CLINICAL GUIDE TO OBSESSIVE COMPULSIVE AND RELATED DISORDERS

Clinical Guide to Obsessive Compulsive and Related Disorders

Jon E. Grant, JD, MD, MPH
Professor of Psychiatry and Behavioral Neuroscience
Pritzker School of Medicine, University of Chicago
Chicago, IL

Samuel R. Chamberlain, MB/BChir, PhD, MRCPsych
Clinical Lecturer
Department of Psychiatry
University of Cambridge, UK

Brian L. Odlaug, MPH
Visiting Researcher
Department of Public Health
Faculty of Health and Medical Sciences
University of Copenhagen
Copenhagen, Denmark

OXFORD
UNIVERSITY PRESS

OXFORD
UNIVERSITY PRESS

Oxford University Press is a department of the University of Oxford. It furthers the University's objective of excellence in research, scholarship, and education by publishing worldwide.

Oxford New York
Auckland Cape Town Dar es Salaam Hong Kong Karachi
Kuala Lumpur Madrid Melbourne Mexico City Nairobi
New Delhi Shanghai Taipei Toronto

With offices in
Argentina Austria Brazil Chile Czech Republic France Greece
Guatemala Hungary Italy Japan Poland Portugal Singapore
South Korea Switzerland Thailand Turkey Ukraine Vietnam

Oxford is a registered trademark of Oxford University Press in the UK and certain other countries.

Published in the United States of America by
Oxford University Press
198 Madison Avenue, New York, NY 10016

Library of Congress Cataloging-in-Publication Data
Grant, Jon E., author.
Clinical Guide to Obsessive Compulsive and Related Disorders / Jon E. Grant, Samuel R. Chamberlain, Brian L. Odlaug
p. ; cm.
Includes bibliographical references.
ISBN 978-0-19-997775-8 (alk. paper)
I. Odlaug, Brian L., author. II. Chamberlain, Samuel, author. III. Title.
[DNLM: 1. Obsessive Compulsive Disorder—therapy—Handbooks. 2. Mental Disorders—Handbooks. 3. Obsessive Compulsive Disorder—diagnosis—Handbooks. WM 34]
RC533
616.85'227—dc23 2013045529

9 8 7 6 5 4 3 2 1
Printed in the United States of America
on acid-free paper

Contents

PART THREE: Special Clinical Considerations

Preface

In writing this guide to Obsessive Compulsive and Related Disorders, instead of providing a detailed and heavy tome, we sought to ask what would be useful for the busy medical student, resident, clinician, psychologist, nurse, and other professional.

In our own careers there have been many times where we had seen a patient with an OC spectrum disorder and wondered what to look out for (co-morbidities not to miss) and what the treatment options were. Often, what followed was a time-consuming search on the Internet, for example, digging out national treatment guidelines or looking through convoluted research databases. This invariably led to more questions, and more time involvement, with work building up in the meantime! Our usual clinical books failed us, providing either no information, or misleading information, on the treatment of these less commonly understood conditions. Even where treatments were mentioned, critical information such as medication starting doses and titration schedules were missing. Where screening tools and disease severity scales were alluded to, they were not included and proved impossible to find within easy reach.

We sought in this book to fill this collective void. It can be read in its entirety as a useful introduction to the OC spectrum, but will also serve as a useful ready reference guide when seeing patients.

We have included many of the key assessment tools for the different conditions in an appendix.

We hope that this book will be useful not only for professionals but also for patients, to better understand their conditions and what treatment options should be available to them.

Disclosure Statements

Dr. Grant is funded by NIMH and the National Center for Responsible Gaming. He receives grant support from Forest Pharmaceuticals and Roche Pharmaceuticals. Dr. Grant receives yearly compensation from Elsevier Publishing for acting as editor-in-chief of the *Journal of Gambling Studies* and receives royalties from Oxford University Press, American Psychiatric Publishing, Inc., Norton Press, and McGraw Hill.

Dr. Chamberlain has received consultancy fees from Cambridge Cognition and P1Vital. He receives compensation from Elsevier Publishing for acting as Associate Editor at *Neuroscience and Biobehavioral Reviews.* Dr. Chamberlain has received speaker fees from Eli Lilly. His research is supported by a grant from the Academy of Medical Sciences (AMS), United Kingdom.

Mr. Odlaug has received grant support from the Trichotillomania Learning Center. He receives consultancy fees from Lundbeck Pharmaceuticals, and royalties from Oxford University Press.

PART ONE

OVERVIEW AND EVALUATION

1

Introduction

Overview of Obsessive Compulsive Disorder

Obsessive Compulsive Disorder (OCD) is characterized by obsessions and/or compulsions. Obsessions are repetitive, intrusive thoughts that are difficult to suppress. Compulsions are repetitive mental or physical rituals that are undertaken either in a stereotyped way (according to rigid rules) or in response to intrusive thoughts. While intrusive thoughts (e.g., "Did I lock the front door?") and compulsions (e.g., double-checking the front door is locked) are fairly common in the background population, in OCD these thoughts and actions occupy at least an hour each day and detract from the ability of the person to engage fully in their daily lives.

People with OCD often only seek help after suffering from the disorder for many years, in some cases being ashamed of their experiences or fearing that they will not be sensitively understood by healthcare professionals. In addition, healthcare professionals do not always screen for OCD and so many are left undiagnosed. This is unfortunate because OCD is treatable, yet chronically untreated symptoms not only are more ingrained (treatment resistant), but also lead to other conditions (e.g., depression).

The most common symptoms in OCD are contamination-related obsessions and cleaning/washing compulsions, but many other types of symptoms exist (see Table 1.1). The variety of symptoms that occur in OCD can present a challenge to clinicians in terms of diagnosis and treatment, there being some evidence that symptoms vary in terms of response to psychological and pharmacological treatments.

TABLE 1.1 Examples of Common Symptoms in OCD

Symptom type	*Examples*
	Obsessions
Contamination-related	Fear that one may be contaminated: - by infections (e.g., sexually transmitted diseases) - by body fluids (urine, semen, feces) - by environmental factors (radiation leakage, dirt on the floor, cleaning products, gasoline)
Sex-related	Recurrent thoughts about: - sexuality (homosexuality, bestiality) - perverse thoughts or impulses (sex acts involving children or family members, sexual violence)
Religion-related	Thoughts about: - heaven/hell, offending god, blasphemy - morality
Control-related	Fears regarding: - acting on impulses (e.g., throwing the baby in boiling water; jumping in front of a train) - shouting out swear words or insults - disturbing intrusive images
Harm-related	Concerns regarding: - being responsible for a terrible outcome (e.g., murder) - endangering loved ones or friends due to lack of care (e.g., dropping the baby)
Perfectionism-related	Intrusive thoughts about: - the need for exactness and symmetry - the need to remember important information - the need for hoarding items that "may some day be useful"

TABLE 1.1 Continued

Symptom type	*Examples*
Superstition-related	Concerns about: - some colors, numbers, or items being "lucky" or "unlucky"
Compulsions	
Washing/ cleaning-related	Repetitive: - hand-washing - bathing (showers/using the bath) - other cleaning (cleaning one's teeth, trimming one's nails) - house chores such as polishing, decontaminating surfaces, or vacuuming
Checking-related	Repeated checking: - that nothing terrible happened (e.g., one didn't kill a pedestrian while driving) - that one did not make a critical mistake - that nothing was forgotten (list writing and checking) - that a particular body part is "okay"
Repetition-related	Recurrent stereotyped: - reading - routines (including sequences of actions being completed a certain number of times in order to be "just right") - body movements / tapping items - collecting of useless items - confessions to others (including healthcare professionals)
Mental compulsion-related	- counting (e.g., to complete a task or prevent some horrible outcome) - praying - canceling out words

OCD is a serious and often disabling psychiatric condition that is under-diagnosed and under-treated. Errors are also made even when treatment is given: one study found that less than half of OCD patients treated with medication received appropriate doses of medication. Left untreated, or treated sub-optimally, OCD is associated with profound impairments in quality of life and functioning, affecting family and home life, relationships, scholastic achievements, and work.

Although some people may experience episodes of OCD that last for a year or two that remit and possibly reappear years later, most individuals, if untreated, have a chronic course of the illness.

Overview of Related Disorders

Improved scientific understanding of OCD (such as understanding its neurobiology, along with co-morbid expression) has led to the idea that this condition represents one of several related disorders. This proposal is recognized in the Diagnostic and Statistical Manual Version 5 (DSM-5): OCD has been moved from the "Anxiety Disorder" section (as in DSM-IV) and now sits in its own category of "Obsessive Compulsive and Related Disorders." For the purposes of this book, we consider the OC Related Disorders to include OCD (the prototype), along with Hoarding Disorder, Body Dysmorphic Disorder (BDD), Hypochondriasis (Illness Anxiety Disorder), Grooming Disorders (Trichotillomania and Excoriation Disorder), and Tic Disorders (Tourette's Disorder, Persistent Tic Disorder, and Provisional Tic Disorder).

Collectively, the OC Related Disorders are indeed "related" from several perspectives: in terms of phenomenology (nature of symptoms), underlying causal factors (genetic and environmental), their tendency to co-occur within individuals (co-morbidity) and families (familiality), and—to some extent—treatment response. While other conditions (such as Binge-Eating Disorder and Pathological Gambling) arguably share parallels with OCD, we do not consider them as OC Related Disorders, because they share less in common with the above-listed conditions.

The hallmark of the OC Related Disorders is the engagement in repetitive functionally impairing habits that are difficult to suppress. Current neurobiological models of the OC Related Disorders emphasize the likely involvement of excessive habit generation from evolutionary ancient parts of the brain (the striatum) coupled with a lack of sufficient top-down control over these habits from cortical regions (especially the frontal lobes).

In *Hoarding Disorder*, individuals accumulate possessions of little use and/or value, and fail to throw them away. Hoarding was classically considered an OCD symptom but more recent work suggests that it may represent a distinct syndrome. In DSM-5, Hoarding Disorder is explicitly distinguished from OCD for the first time. Hoarding is usually ego-syntonic, that is, the symptoms are acceptable to the individual and are undertaken "in harmony" with the person's sense of will. In this way it is quite different from most cases of OCD, where symptoms are ego-dystonic: the thoughts and behaviors in archetypal OCD are distressing to the person's ego and they attempt to resist but often fail to do so. Hoarding Disorder is often more difficult to treat than OCD and may begin earlier in life with stronger genetic influences.

Body Dysmorphic Disorder (BDD) is characterized by a preoccupation with a slight or imagined defect in appearance. This preoccupation frequently is of delusional intensity: that is, the person is convinced that their flaw is "hideous" or "disfiguring" despite the fact that others may see little if anything wrong with the person. People with BDD engage in rituals including checking themselves in the mirror, trying to mask the perceived defect (using makeup or covering up using clothing), or over-exercising. In BDD, individuals may seek the attention of surgeons with a view to correcting the perceived defect or may attempt to address the perceived defect themselves using dangerous "do-it-yourself" home surgical interventions. It is important to note that suicidality is a particular concern in BDD, with higher rates of suicide attempts and completed suicide, than seen in other OC Related Conditions.

Hypochondriasis, now known as "Illness Anxiety Disorder" in DSM-5, is associated with excessive preoccupation with the idea that one has (or is likely to develop) a serious physical illness. People with Hypochondriasis habitually and repetitively seek-out general practitioners and other medical clinicians due to these concerns. They are likely to request various medical tests but—to the stress of the clinician—are seldom reassured by normal results (quite the contrary). Health providers can paradoxically contribute to the persistence of this disabling condition by "feeding into" it with their own anxieties and repeated investigations. People with Hypochondriasis will seldom seek out psychiatric help since they are unlikely to appreciate the psychological nature of their experiences without this being sensitively explained (psychoeducation). Nonetheless they should be encouraged to see a psychiatrist or other mental health professional.

Grooming Disorders (Trichotillomania, Excoriation [Skin Picking] Disorder) are especially poorly recognized as such by professionals and by sufferers. Affected individuals repeatedly pull out their own hair, pick at their skin, and/or bite down their nails. While these types of behavior are common in society, in Grooming Disorders the habits get out of control and lead to functional impairment. These symptoms not only impact negatively on the individual due to the *time* they occupy, but can also lead to considerable physical disfigurement, with concomitant loss of self-esteem, and avoidance of sport, social activities, and intimate relationships. The habits have potentially serious physical consequences: for example, excessive skin picking can lead to skin infection and sepsis; ingesting hair can lead to gastrointestinal obstruction (a surgical emergency). Individuals may avoid contact with others and use cosmetic products or clothing (such as scarves or hats) to prevent others from noticing the disfigurement.

In *Tic Disorders* (Tourette's Disorder, Persistent Tic Disorder, and Provisional Tic Disorder), patients experience repetitive, rapid, non-rhythmic motor movements and/or vocalizations (these can be simple guttural noises or, less commonly, actual words). A patient may have various tic symptoms over time. Although tics can include almost any muscle group or vocalization, certain tics, such as eye blinking or throat clearing, are common. Tics are generally experienced as involuntary but can be voluntarily suppressed for varying lengths of time. In addition, tics can be either simple (i.e., short duration, such as milliseconds, and can include eye blinking, shoulder shrugging, throat clearing, sniffing, and grunting) or complex (i.e., longer duration, such as seconds, and include a combination of simple tics such as simultaneous head turning and shoulder shrugging). Tics are often seen in children and do not necessarily constitute "a disorder" or require treatment unless they become a problem for the individual. In fact, many individuals with mild to moderate tics experience no distress or impairment in functioning and may even be unaware of their tics. Less commonly, tics disrupt daily functioning and result in social isolation, being bullied by peers, inability to work or to go to school, and low quality of life. Rare complications of Tourette's Disorder include physical injury, such as eye injury (from hitting oneself in the face), and orthopedic and neurological injury (e.g., disc disease related to forceful head and neck movements).

Epidemiology and Etiology

The prevalence of OCD has been well-studied in population-wide surveys across the globe: these studies show that OCD occurs in 1–3% of the population at some point in life ("lifetime prevalence"), that OCD cuts across cultures and countries, and that men and women are similarly at risk of being affected. Lifetime prevalence and epidemiological features of the other OC Spectrum Disorders are less well studied. Key epidemiological characteristics of the OC Related Disorders are summarized below (Table 1.2). It should be noted that there is considerable variation in the course of these conditions, which is likely to be affected by age of onset, duration of untreated disease, availability of optimal treatments, compliance with treatment, and a balance between predisposing-persisting versus resilience-mitigating factors.

TABLE 1.2 Prevalence, Course, and Variance of OCD and Related Disorders

Disorder	*Lifetime prevalence estimate*	*Gender distribution*	*Average age of symptom onset*	*Typical course*
OCD	1–3%	M = F	Bimodal distribution with peak age 10y and in early adulthood	Often persists despite treatment into middle-age; long-term may resolve on its own
Hoarding Disorder	0.5–2%	M > F	10y	Often persists lifelong without treatment
Body Dysmorphic Disorder	1%	M = F	17y	Likely to be chronic without treatment
Illness Anxiety Disorder (Hypochondriasis)	1–5%	M > F	25–40y	Variable. Likely to be chronic, especially in individuals with co-morbid anxiety and depression
Trichotillomania	0.5–2%	M < F	12–13y	Very early onset may resolve spontaneously but otherwise likely to follow relapsing-remitting course into adulthood
Skin Picking Disorder	0.5–2%	M < F	12–13y	Very early onset may resolve spontaneously but otherwise likely to follow relapsing-remitting course into adulthood
Tic Disorders	0.5–5%	M > F	6–7y (phonic tics develop later)	Often resolves by adulthood

In most cases of OCD and Related Disorders there is no single or simplistic cause. A good way of explaining this is to state that although the cause is unknown, there are likely to be many factors (e.g., genetic vulnerability, unique biology, developmental/environmental issues, etc.) each conferring an element of risk.

Many parents with OCD or a related disorder often want to know if they can pass along their illness to their children. It is therefore important to know something about the genetics of these disorders. The influence of genetics over OC disorders has been investigated using family studies. For example, it has been found that first-degree relatives of people with OCD have a 3–4 times greater risk of developing OCD themselves, as compared to controls. This risk ratio is probably similar for the other OC Related Disorders. Environmental factors are also very important but not well characterized.

Another way of understanding OC Related Disorders is to consider underlying brain processes. The main techniques that have been used to study these conditions are:

- *Cognitive tests.* Volunteers undertake paper-and-pencil or computerized tests that are dependent on particular brain circuitry and neurochemical systems. Comparison is made between cognitive abilities in people with OCD and people without OCD, and relationships with symptoms are explored.
- *Structural brain scans* (computerized tomography [CT] and magnetic resonance imaging [MRI]). Volunteers enter a brain scanner and undertake one or more scans. Measures of average "brain structure" are extracted and then compared between different groups (e.g., people with OCD and matched control volunteers).
- *Functional brain scans* (functional magnetic resonance imaging [fMRI]). Volunteers enter a brain scanner and undertake one or more scans capable of measuring brain oxygen use/metabolic activity (for example, volunteers might undertake a test of memory function while lying in the scanner by

watching a computer screen and making responses with a button box). Different techniques, such as positron emission tomography (PET), are more costly but have started to be used to explore brain receptors and chemical transporter systems.

The above techniques have identified differences between groups of patients versus healthy volunteers in research studies, but have yet to be shown to be sensitive or useful on an individual subject level. Therefore, there is currently no clinical indication for routine cognitive testing and brain scanning in patients with OC Related Disorders, except in cases where organic pathology is suspected (e.g., suspicion of a dementing illness; e.g., patient shows neurologic abnormalities on clinical examination).

Collectively, of the OC family of disorders, OCD and Tic Disorders are the best studied from the perspective of underlying brain processes. These conditions have been associated with cognitive difficulties (difficulty suppressing inappropriate responses) along with abnormalities in brain structure (grey matter [neurone cell bodies] and white matter [neuronal connections]) and function (under- and over-activation of brain circuitry during cognitive challenge and symptom provocation). Most commonly affected brain regions across these disorders include the ventral and dorsal striatum (nucleus accumbens, involved in reward; putamen/caudate, involved in habit repetition) and the frontal cortices (especially dorsolateral and orbitofrontal). Critically, these abnormalities are not generally detectable on an individual-by-individual basis and rather represent crude averaged differences between patients and volunteers without the given disorder being studied. Researchers may look back in future years and consider these efforts simplistic. Intriguingly, some cognitive problems and their brain correlates exist in people at risk of OC Related Disorders even before the symptoms have developed, suggesting that they may represent a predisposing (rather than directly causative) influence. The Table 1.3 highlights key neurobiological findings across the OC Family: it should be noted that there do appear to be important

TABLE 1.3 Neurobiological Findings from Neuroimaging and Neuropsychological Tests

Disorder	*Cognitive findings*	*Structural brain findings*	*Functional brain findings*
OCD	Deficits across a range of cognitive domains including attentional flexibility, inhibitory control, working memory, and executive planning; decision-making usually intact	Increased grey matter in the basal ganglia (mainly putamen and caudate) coupled with reduced grey matter in bilateral frontal and anterior cingulate cortices. Abnormal integrity of white matter tracts connecting these regions	OCD symptom-provocation is associated with activation of distinct neural regions (especially caudate nucleus; orbitofrontal and anterior cingulate cortices). Some evidence that different OCD symptom types involve different brain regions. Under-activation of key neural regions during cognitive challenge (such as under-activation of orbitofrontal and parietal cortices during tests of flexible responding; such as reduced recruitment of caudate and precuneus during executive planning)
Hoarding Disorder	Strikingly similar deficits to those found in OCD (as above)	Not well studied. Hoarding-OCD appears similar to findings in non-hoarding OCD (as above)	Symptom-provocation is associated with disproportionate activation in neural regions such as the bilateral orbitofrontal and anterior cingulate cortices (appears to be narrower range of regions than those activating abnormally in OCD generally)

(continued)

TABLE 1.3 Continued

Disorder	*Cognitive findings*	*Structural brain findings*	*Functional brain findings*
Body Dysmorphic Disorder (BDD)	Some evidence for deficits in working memory and executive planning; other functions not yet examined	Not well studied; small sample sizes only. Some evidence for reduced grey matter in orbitofrontal and anterior cingulate versus controls	Evidence of abnormal brain activation when viewing faces (greater activity in left prefrontal cortex and temporal lobe than controls; also in caudate)
Illness Anxiety Disorder (Hypochondriasis)	Not yet known	Not yet known	Paucity of data. Under-activation of caudate and precuneus during executive planning, similar to OCD
Trichotillomania	More selective cognitive problems compared to OCD: most commonly affected function is inhibitory control. Some evidence for problems with working memory and cognitive flexibility, depending on sample studied	Increased grey matter densities in the left striatum, left amygdalo-hippocampal formation, and multiple (including cingulate, supplementary motor, and frontal) cortical regions bilaterally. Abnormal integrity of white matter tracts connecting these regions	Not yet known

Skin Picking Disorder	More selective cognitive problems compared to OCD: most commonly affected function is inhibitory control	Remarkably similar findings to those in Trichotillomania (overlapping neural abnormalities)	Not yet known
Tic Disorders	More selective cognitive problems compared to OCD: inhibitory control appears to be most affected, but not in all studies	Considerable heterogeneity in terms of grey matter findings: some evidence for abnormal grey matter in caudate and hippocampus. Abnormal white matter integrity in distributed tracts including those involved in somatosensory and motor processing	fMRI implicates supplementary motor area activation in premonitory sensations/urges and activation of regions such as somatosensory and premotor cortices in the generation of tics. Some evidence for elevated task-related activations (especially prefrontal cortex) on inhibitory control tasks

differences between conditions, which may account for why treatment approaches for them differ as will be seen in subsequent chapters.

Diagnosis and Co-morbidity

In diagnosing OCD and Related Disorders, the reader should give due consideration to the specific criteria laid down, either in the Diagnostic and Statistical Manual (DSM), or in the International Classification of Diseases (ICD). For convenience, the diagnostic criteria for each condition are listed in the individual book chapters, along with details of recommended screening tools and methods for assessing disease severity and treatment response. Proper diagnosis ensures a common language for clinicians.

Be mindful of co-morbidities, the most common of which are listed in the individual chapters for each OC condition. Co-morbidities should be regarded as the norm for most patients rather than the exception. Many people experience intrusive repetitive thoughts that must be carefully distinguished from obsessions. For example, people with depression often have recurrent depressive ruminations (thoughts of failure and catastrophizing), people with (hypo)mania experience racing ideas (e.g., grandiose thoughts), and people with General Anxiety Disorder may have excessive worries about the future. Unlike these types of intrusive thoughts, obsessions are usually experienced as senseless/inappropriate, and are to some degree resisted by the sufferer. The presence of intrusive thoughts related to food or body image should prompt the clinician to think about the possibility of BDD or an eating disorder.

Different types of compulsions can be distinguished from each other by considering the phenomenology (descriptive nature of the symptom) along with antecedents and consequences. In OCD, compulsions are usually undertaken to reduce distress (anxiety) triggered by obsessions, while tics and repetitive grooming tend to happen without obsessive antecedents. Complex tics are unlikely to be present if there are no simple tics. People with OCD and Tic Disorders are likely to recognize their compulsions as being unwanted and negative (ego-dystonic), while checking in BDD and the keeping of possessions in Hoarding Disorder are unlikely to be recognized in this way (ego-syntonic).

Treatment

The treatment of OCD and Related Disorders in specific individuals should be determined by (1) the scientific evidence, (2) patient factors, (3) service factors, and (4) ethical considerations.

In this book, we have sought to distil the evidence base and provide clear guidelines on treatment for the various disorders. In terms of medication options, various jurisdictions have approved certain medications for the treatment of OCD and related disorders. In addition, scientific evidence may support non-approved medication options as well.

Patient factors that should be considered as a general principle when determining treatment choice include the nature and severity of symptoms, co-morbid medical and psychiatric conditions, any past treatments received and response to these, current medications, and patient/family preferences.

Availability of treatments, and waiting lists, also place pragmatic restraints on what can be offered, and this is likely to vary considerably depending on geographical location and context (service factors), which are often largely outside of the healthcare professional's control.

Ethical considerations are always relevant, namely: non-maleficence (do no harm), beneficence (do good), and justice (appropriate and fair allocation of resources). In practice for clinicians, this means weighing the pros and cons of a given treatment and being sure to discuss these with the patient to facilitate informed decision-making.

Key References

- Blanco C, Olfson M, Stein DJ, et al. Treatment of obsessive-compulsive disorder by U.S. psychiatrists. J Clin Psychiatry. 2006 Jun;67(6):946–51.
- Castle DJ, Phillips KA. Obsessive compulsive spectrum of disorders: a defensible construct? Aust N Z J Psychiatry. 2006 Feb;40(2):114–20.
- Veldhuis J, Dieleman JP, Wohlfarth T, Storosum JG, van Den Brink W, Sturkenboom MC, Denys D. Incidence and prevalence of "diagnosed OCD" in a primary care, treatment seeking, population. Int J Psychiatry Clin Pract. 2012 Jun;16(2):85–92.

2

Evaluation and Treatment Planning

General Aspects of an Evaluation

A comprehensive clinical evaluation is necessary for deciding upon appropriate treatment. The evaluation for someone with obsessive compulsive disorder (OCD) does not differ greatly from that used for any general psychiatric evaluation, and the principles described here can be similarly applied to other OC disorders.

The evaluation needs to focus on the history of present illness, co-occurring mental and physical health issues (see each disorder for the specific co-morbidities), a review of medical and mental health systems, medication, family and social histories, and current mental status examination.

Other general questions that help with the assessment of OCD and related disorders also apply to psychiatric evaluations:

- What prompted the person to present for an assessment now?
- What are the expectations of the patient?
- What is the patient's knowledge concerning their condition?
- How has the condition affected the person's life? How has the condition affected other people in the patient's life?
- Are there conditions, both medical and psychological, that co-occur with the presenting issue?
- What previous treatment approaches has the person tried? If they have received previous treatment, what was their feeling about these treatments?

During the evaluation, it is also appropriate to tell the patient:

- What you see the goal of treatment being;
- How you plan to measure change during treatment; and
- What you expect of the patient

Suicide Risk

Evaluate suicide risk in all patients. Individuals with OCD and related disorders may become overwhelmed by their obsessions and their inability to function normally, prompting suicidal ideation and behaviors. Some OC related disorders, such as Body Dysmorphic Disorder (BDD), show very high rates of suicidality.

OCD Patient Interview

Content of the Obsessions

Clinicians need to remember that OCD is not simply about contamination and washing compulsions. There are numerous variations of OCD and, in many cases, unless specifically asked, the patient will not discuss certain obsessive thoughts. This is particularly true for the "taboo" obsessions of aggression, sex, and religion. Patients report feeling as if they will be judged by the clinician or even reported to the police for having such thoughts and then not treated if they divulge these obsessions.

The OCD interview starts with:

1) Ask the patient whether they have any thoughts that are intrusive, troubling, and that they cannot stop.
2) In addition, the clinician then needs to ask about any behaviors that are performed over and over again and that interfere with the person's life or are distressing.

If the person does not fully understand the initial questions or seems reticent about answering, a follow-up question might be something such as:

"Many people have recurrent thoughts about any number of troubling ideas—contamination by germs, needing to have everything symmetrical, needing things "just right," thoughts about their health, or even more troubling thoughts about sacrilegious, violent, or sexual behaviors—and they cannot seem to control these thoughts. Do you have any issues similar to these?"

Even when the patient endorses one particular theme of their obsessions, it is important to ask about the others as well. Many people with OCD have multiple obsessive thoughts and although one may be their primary obsession, it is important to assess and be aware of the others as well. Some people will report that the obsessive themes change over time resulting in the clinician feeling as if there is success when one obsession is gone without knowing another obsessive thought has become more significant.

If you feel you cannot remember all of the forms of OCD (of which there are many), going through the Yale-Brown Obsessive Compulsive Scale Symptom Checklist will allow for a thorough assessment of all types of OCD.

Details about OCD

Other questions that are clinically important to ask about OCD include:

- At what age did obsessive symptoms begin? (OCD generally starts before age 25 years; a late onset of OCD [>50 years of age] should make the clinician consider other possible diagnoses, such as neurological conditions / central nervous system pathologies)
- Have you experienced any period of time without obsessive thoughts?

- What, if anything, makes the OCD better or worse (e.g., stress, poor night's sleep, alcohol/drugs, exercise, etc.)?
- Does anyone in your family have similar symptoms?

If the patient reports that previous therapy was not helpful, it is important to ask detailed questions about their therapy to determine if they received adequate cognitive behavioral therapy (CBT) using exposure ritual response prevention. Many patients may think they have received appropriate therapy but upon closer scrutiny, it may become apparent that the therapy was inadequate (e.g., patient failed to do homework exercises; therapy did not incorporate appropriate exposure; therapy terminated after too few sessions).

Differentiating Obsessions in OCD from Other Conditions

Depressive ruminations. The clinician needs to be able to differentiate obsessions in OCD from the depressive ruminations seen in mood disorders. When asked about constant intrusive thoughts, the depressed person with ruminations will also answer affirmatively. The clinician can usually separate these concepts by asking whether the content of the obsessive thoughts involves negative self-assessment, castigating oneself about the past, or generally about low self-worth—all general symptoms of depressive ruminations. In addition, the person will likely meet other criteria for depression. Also, the clinician should ask the patient whether these thoughts occur only in the context of the other depressive symptoms. This is again evidence for depressive ruminations if they answer affirmatively. It should be noted that OCD (and related conditions) often co-occur with depression and that patients may well meet diagnostic criteria for both depression and an OC related disorder. In these cases, OCD patients will meet criteria for depression (and experience a number of ruminations to do with negative self worth and failure), along with more generalized intrusive thoughts (such as relating to contamination).

Anxious worries. Generally anxious people may also endorse the question of intrusive thoughts. The distinction between general anxiety and OCD, however, is that usually anxiety-related thoughts relate to real-life events such as employment, financial, or relationship issues. In addition, there are no compulsive behaviors that coincide with general anxiety thoughts.

Psychotic ruminations. Although individuals with OCD may intermittently lack insight into their beliefs (e.g., they feel convinced that they can contract HIV from the doorknob), this lack of insight usually fluctuates. In addition, they do not have other psychotic symptoms or other delusional beliefs outside of their obsession. This is unlike schizophrenia, in which the person may have other psychotic symptoms such as hallucinations and there is rarely any insight unless treated.

Weight obsessions. If the person endorses intrusive thoughts, the clinician should ask whether the thoughts are about weight and fear of obesity. The thoughts seen in eating disorders often look very similar to those of OCD. Since treatments for eating disorders and OCD differ, however, making this distinction is important.

Perfectionism. This may be the most difficult topic when the person expresses problems with not meeting a vision of perfection that they feel they should. They will endorse intrusive thoughts but they generally like the thoughts, even though they may feel frustrated with not achieving all they desire. The trait of obsessive perfectionism may be indicative of Obsessive Compulsive Personality Disorder (OCPD). If this trait is endorsed, the clinician should screen for the other symptoms of OCPD. If OCPD is present, these thoughts are unlikely to remit, and it is not even clear that should be the goal. Instead, the goal is most properly conceptualized as reducing the intensity of the thoughts to allow less distress for the person, not to eliminate traits that in fact may be advantageous to some degree.

Severity of the OCD Symptoms

When examining someone with OCD, it is important to establish a baseline severity so that improvement or lack thereof can be assessed in subsequent visits. The clinician could use a standardized severity instrument (e.g., the Yale-Brown Obsessive Compulsive Scale [YBOCS]) which rates the severity of both obsessions and compulsions. In lieu of such an instrument, however, there are some basic questions (based on the YBOCS) that offer important severity information.

- In general for the past week, how much time in an average day do the obsessions occupy?
- In general for the past week, how much time in an average day do the compulsive behaviors occupy?
- Describe how the obsessions and compulsions interfere with your life currently.
- Describe the distress the obsessions and compulsions currently cause you.

These questions should then be asked at each visit to monitor symptom change.

Standardized Instruments

There are standardized instruments to assist with the diagnosis of OCD and related disorders and there are instruments used to assess symptom severity.

Diagnostic Instruments

OCD and other psychiatric disorders can be reliability diagnosed using the Structured Clinical Interview for DSM (SCID). This is a clinician-administered instrument that may take up to 90 minutes if screening for all psychiatric disorders, but it provides information on both current and lifetime disorders. However, the module for OCD can be used on its own in clinical practice to make a reliable and valid diagnosis of OCD.

The Mini-International Neuropsychiatric Interview can also be used to diagnose OCD and certain other psychiatric disorders. The instrument mostly assesses current disorders, not lifetime. The OCD questions could be used on their own to help with the diagnosis.

The Yale-Brown Obsessive Compulsive Scale Symptom Checklist is not a diagnostic instrument but once the diagnosis of OCD is made, this instrument can provide the clinician with a thorough assessment of every obsessive thought and compulsion that the person has or had in the past.

Severity Instruments

The Yale-Brown Obsessive Compulsive Scale (Y-BOCS: see Appendix C) is a 10-item clinician-administered scale which has become the most widely used scale to assess symptom severity. The Y-BOCS is comprised of 5 questions regarding obsessive thoughts during the past week and 5 questions concerning compulsive behaviors during the past week. Each question is scored from 0=no symptoms to 4=extreme symptoms. A total score of 0–7 is subclinical OCD, 8–15 mild OCD, 16–23 moderate OCD, 24–31 severe OCD, and 32–40 is extreme OCD. An improvement of 35% or more on the Y-BOCS during treatment has been considered a clinically meaningful response and translates generally into better overall functioning.

The Obsessive Compulsive Inventory Revised (OCI-R: Appendix C) is a 42-item scale composed of 7 subscales: Washing, Checking, Doubting, Ordering, Obsessing (i.e., having obsessional thoughts), Hoarding, and Mental Neutralizing. Each item is rated on a 5-point (0–4) scale of symptom distress. Mean scores are calculated for each of the seven subscales and an overall mean "distress" score is calculated. Each score is presented as a mean out of a possible maximum of "4" with lower scores meaning less severe symptoms. A total score of 42 or more, or a mean score of 2.5 or more in any of the subscales, suggests the presence of OCD.

Note: The OCI is not meant to be diagnostic but can help the clinician to determine the severity of OCD symptoms.

The Maudsley Obsessive Compulsive Inventory (MOCI) is a 30-question, true/false format, patient-report questionnaire consisting of 4 subscales: checking, washing/cleaning compulsions, slowness, and doubting. Total "true" responses are added to obtain a total score. The scale is split between 15 obsessive questions and 15 compulsive questions but does not cover all such symptoms. As such, the MOCI can assess for certain but not all obsessive or compulsive symptoms.

The Leyton Obsessional Inventory (LOI) is a 69-question, self-report instrument designed to assess for obsessional symptoms and traits. 46 questions are designed to assess for symptoms of OCD and 23 questions target OC personality traits. For each item the patient endorses, he or she completes a 5-point Likert scale showing his or her level of resistance to that specific symptom or trait as well as a 4-point interference scale measuring the extent to which that symptom or trait interferes with daily activities.

Family Evaluation

If the patient is willing to allow you to talk with family, it is strongly recommended. Family members can provide important information regarding overall functioning and change in functioning.

The family also needs to be assessed for their knowledge about OCD and its treatment. Most families have limited if any knowledge about OCD. Education about OCD may allow family members to be more understanding of the patient and not so easily frustrated. Many family members shame patients hoping that it will "snap them out of it" but this only makes OCD, self-esteem, and depression worse.

Lack of education on the family's part may also have resulted in them allowing the compulsions to occur and, in turn, fuel obsessive thoughts. Part of the treatment approach will involve educating family members about OCD and the importance of not indulging the OCD symptoms. This may result in them not being able to provide reassurance when asked by the patient (a common compulsion) and allowing the OCD to control (e.g., family members may allow the person to spend hours in the bathroom washing even when they are inconvenienced).

Medical Evaluation

A variety of medical conditions are associated with symptoms that resemble obsessions and compulsions. These conditions, however, are rarely the cause of the OCD symptoms except in certain cases. The clinician may consider a medical workup when the OCD (1) has onset after the age of approximately 40, or (2) is temporally associated with recent seizures, head trauma, or new neurological symptoms.

Multiple medical conditions have been associated with OCD but these have been only in case reports and details are often not available. Table 2.1 lists key pathologies along with potential diagnostic tests and interventions.

Medical Work-Up

OCD and related disorders are still largely diagnosed through a careful clinical evaluation. In the majority of cases, there is no need for laboratory or neurodiagnostic work-ups. In the case of an atypical representation or a presentation of OCD with associated new-onset neurological symptoms, further medical work-up may be appropriate.

Treatment Planning

Treatment planning is based on a careful clinical evaluation. The treatment plan should be tailored to the patient's needs, preferences, capacities, situation, and history.

Therapy and/or Medication

For the patient with mild to moderate OCD, a combination of exposure response prevention therapy plus a serotonin reuptake inhibitor (SRI) (i.e., a special class of antidepressant medications which include clomipramine, fluoxetine, paroxetine, sertraline, citalopram, escitalopram, and fluvoxamine) is a reasonable initial strategy. The patient may prefer one of these treatment options instead of another. Either could be effective on its own. The person could begin with one approach and add the other if only partial response is achieved with the initial treatment option. If the mild to moderate OCD patient also has depression, then using an SRI with therapy may be preferred.

If the patient has moderate to severe OCD and the obsessions prevent the person from taking part completely with therapy, an SRI may be a useful starting point to decrease symptoms enough that the person can take advantage of therapy.

Treatment Planning for Co-occurring Disorders

Depression: If the person has significant co-occurring depression with their OCD, both medication and psychotherapy would be appropriate. In that case, a therapeutic approach that includes exposure and response prevent (ERP) but also eclectic enough to include emotional regulation, social skill training, and interpersonal dynamics could be more beneficial than someone rigidly adhering to ERP only.

Substance Use Disorders: In the case of a patient with OCD and Substance Use Disorders, the person may first need detoxification from the substance with some abstinence prior to undergoing ERP for the OCD.

Bipolar Disorder: When bipolar disorder co-occurs with OCD, medications to stabilize mood (e.g., lithium, anti-epileptics) may be needed prior to treatment of the OCD. Given that some uncertainty exists around SRIs inducing hypomania or mania, the first-line of treatment after mood stabilization should be ERP.

TABLE 2.1 Medical Conditions Associated with OCD

Pathology	*Description*	*Investigations*	*Potential interventions*
Infections	Certain infections have been associated with OCD-like symptoms, notably HIV, and Group A beta-hemolytic streptococcal infection	Blood work-up including viral screen, bacteriology, immune status. Brain imaging for HIV	Treatment of underlying pathology with antiretroviral medications (HIV), or antibiotics (streptococcal infection). OCD symptoms can respond to SRIs. Plasmaphoresis and intravenous immunoglobulins are used for PANDAS (see PANDAS section)
Seizures	Partial complex, frontal, and tonic-clinic seizures have all been associated with OCD symptoms	Extensive blood workup including electrolytes, bone profile, liver function tests. Head imaging. Consider possible contribution of prescribed medications, use of alcohol, and illicit substances	Treatment approach unclear. May respond to anti-epileptic medications or SRIs, although clomipramine should be avoided due to lowering of the seizure threshold

(continued)

TABLE 2.1 Continued

Pathology	*Description*	*Investigations*	*Potential interventions*
Head injury	Cases of OCD have been associated with head injury resulting in loss of consciousness	Diagnostic investigations are usually not very revealing	May respond to SRIs
Cerebrovascular infarcts	Infarcts of the right frontal, caudate nuclei, and right putamen areas have all been associated with older age of OCD onset	Consider cardiovascular risk factors that are modifiable (check fasting lipid profile). Brain imaging	The treatment of the OCD symptoms is unclear as some evidence suggests that SRIs may not be effective
Parkinson's Disease	Individuals with Parkinson's disease who are taking dopamine agonists may develop punding behavior that mimics OCD symptoms	N/A	Decreasing or discontinuing the dopamine agonist may eliminate the punding behavior. Since the patient may need some dopamine agonist therapy, however, lowering the dose or changing the medication should be performed before stopping medication completely

Medications/ Drugs	Prescribed and illicit stimulants (e.g., cocaine, amphetamine) have been associated with stereotyped repetitive behaviors and appear to be associated with skin picking and worsening of Trichotillomania (Hair Pulling Disorder) in some people. There is not good evidence, however, that these substances result in obsessive thoughts or are associated with OCD	Detailed medication history and sensitive screening for illicit drug use (including urine toxicology)	Consider reducing prescribed dose of stimulant medication if clinically appropriate to do so. Support patients in reducing intake of illicit substances and treat these addictions rigorously

Severe OCD Cases

In severe cases of OCD, in-patient or partial hospitalization programs may be necessary, and rarely psychosurgery may be utilized. Please see the section on these interventions elsewhere.

Key References

- Benito K, Storch EA. Assessment of obsessive compulsive disorder: review and future directions. Expert Rev Neurother. 2011 Feb;11(2):287–98.
- Figee M, Wielaard I, Mazaheri A, Denys D. Neurosurgical targets for compulsivity: what can we learn from acquired brain lesions? Neurosci Biobehav Rev. 2013 Mar;37(3):328–39.
- Fineberg NA, Krishnaiah RB, Moberg J, O'Doherty C. Clinical screening for obsessive compulsive and related disorders. Isr J Psychiatry Relat Sci. 2008;45(3):151–63.

PART TWO

OBSESSIVE COMPULSIVE AND RELATED DISORDERS

3

Obsessive Compulsive Disorder

Clinical Description

The hallmark of obsessive compulsive disorder (OCD) is the presence of obsessions and/or compulsions. Obsessions are repetitive and intrusive persistent ideas, thoughts, urges, or images experienced as intrusive and inappropriate and that cause marked anxiety or distress. Examples include fears of germs and contamination. Obsessions are not pleasurable or experienced as voluntary: they are intrusive and unwanted and cause marked distress or anxiety in most individuals. The individual attempts to ignore or suppress these obsessions or to neutralize them with another thought or action (e.g., performing a compulsion).

Compulsions are repetitive and intentional behaviors or mental acts performed in response to obsessions or according to certain rules that must be applied rigidly. Examples include repetitive hand washing and ritualistic checking. Compulsions are meant to neutralize or reduce the person's discomfort or prevent a dreaded event or situation. The rituals are not connected in a realistic way to the event or situation or are clearly excessive. Obsessive compulsive disorder has a lifetime prevalence of 1.6–3% and comprises one of the top causes of global disability according to the World Health Organization.

Diagnosis

The DSM-5 Diagnostic Criteria for Obsessive Compulsive Disorder require the presence of obsessions, compulsions, or both.

"Obsessions" are defined by recurrent thoughts, urges, or images that are experienced, at some time, as intrusive and unwanted, and that in most individuals cause marked anxiety or distress. In addition, the person attempts to ignore or suppress such thoughts, urges, or images, or to neutralize them with some other thought or action (i.e., by performing a compulsion).

"Compulsions" are characterized by repetitive behaviors (e.g., hand washing, ordering, checking) or mental acts (e.g., praying, counting) that the person feels driven to perform in response to an obsession. The goal of these compulsive behaviors is to prevent or reduce anxiety or distress, or prevent some feared outcome.

The DSM-5 criteria also require that the obsessions or compulsions are time-consuming (e.g., take more than 1 hour per day) or cause significant distress or psychosocial impairment.

The symptoms of obsessive compulsive disorder cannot be solely attributable to the effects of a substance (e.g., a drug of abuse, a medication) or another medical condition.

The DSM-5 further allows for specifiers to characterize the level of insight the person has about their disorder. They might have good or fair insight if able to recognize that their beliefs are definitely or probably not true, poor insight if they think their beliefs are probably true, or no insight in the case where they believe the thoughts are true. If the person has a current or past history of a Tic Disorder they receive the specifier "tic-related" for their OCD.

Clinical Features

Obsessions and compulsions present in an infinite number of ways focusing on a number of themes: contamination, aggression, harm avoidance, distasteful sexual thoughts, religious or moral issues, a need to know things, a need for symmetry, to name only a few. Contamination fears are the most common obsessive thought, and cleaning and checking are the most commonly reported compulsions. Multiple obsessions and compulsions are common. In addition, the theme of the obsessions and compulsions may change over the course of the illness.

The mean age at onset of OCD is 19.5 years, and 25% of cases start by age 14 years. Onset after age 35 years is unusual but does occur. Males have an earlier age at onset than females: nearly 25% of males have an OCD onset before age 10 years. The onset of symptoms is typically gradual, however, acute onset has also been reported.

How OCD Differs from Normal Behavior

Everyone obsesses about some event from time to time. The diagnosis of OCD, however, generally requires that obsessive thoughts occur for more than 1 hour each day. In addition, obsessions of OCD do not suddenly start and stop with a specific event. If you are worried about a loved one being treated for cancer you may think about the possible outcomes for more than 1 hour each day but after the cancer enters remission, you probably reduce your thinking or stop worrying about it. Someone with OCD may reduce their obsessions after an event but they will generally focus on some new topic at the same level of intensity.

Various Forms of OCD

Although many people know about contamination obsessions and washing compulsions, there are many variations of OCD. It may be helpful to have the patient complete the Yale-Brown Obsessive Compulsive Scale Symptom Checklist, which lists dozens of possible obsessions and compulsions. Patients often do not realize that certain thoughts they have are OCD.

Some common obsessions include:

Taboo: These obsessive thoughts focus on sex, sacrilegious thoughts, and/or violence. Many patients will not mention these unless specifically asked. An example might be thoughts of having sex with children while in church and then killing them. In response to these obsessive thoughts, the patient believes he is a horrible person and so may worry excessively and ask for forgiveness from a priest or other religious leader.

Just Right: These obsessions focus on not doing things correctly or a feeling of incompleteness which thereby negatively affects others or the patient. The corresponding compulsion may be a need to recheck excessively. Checking financial records dozens of times or arranging items in an exact order are examples of compulsions possibly prompted by just right obsessionality.

Symmetry: These obsessions focus on having things done in balance, touching things in certain fashion to balance things, etc. Corresponding compulsions may include lining up or putting objects in a certain symmetrical order or color matching.

Co-morbidity

Major Depressive Disorder: Major depression is the most common co-morbid condition in OCD. In fact, approximately 63% of individuals with OCD will have depression. Individuals with co-morbid depression might display more sadness, anhedonia, and other depressive symptoms. Individuals who are depressed may exhibit depressive ruminations—that is, constant thoughts about mistakes they made in life, paths not taken, etc. These may look like obsessions but are, in fact, part of the depressive disorder. Clinical trial data indicate that depressive symptoms respond more rapidly to SRI treatment than obsessive compulsive symptoms. The reasons for this are not well understood but likely relate to different involvement of the serotonin system in the two disorders.

Hoarding Disorder: Hoarding is the acquisition of and failure to discard a large number of possessions. The patient also experiences substantial distress or impairment in the ability to use living areas of the home for their intended purposes. Hoarding is surprisingly common and is potentially seriously disabling. Although significant hoarding has recently been shown to occur in 2–5% of the general population, the rate of hoarding among individuals with OCD ranges from 25% to 30%.

Anxiety Disorders: Many adults with OCD have a lifetime diagnosis of an anxiety disorder (76%; e.g., Panic Disorder, social anxiety disorder, generalized anxiety disorder, specific phobia). Onset of OCD is usually later than for most anxiety disorders (with the exception of separation anxiety disorder) and post-traumatic stress disorder (PTSD).

Obsessive Compulsive Personality Disorder: Co-morbid Obsessive Compulsive Personality Disorder is common in individuals with OCD (e.g., ranging from 23% to 32%). Obsessive Compulsive Personality Disorder is marked by rigid perfectionism or morality with interpersonal difficulties. While OCD and Obsessive Compulsive Personality Disorder are often confused in common parlance, they often occur independently of each other and they have very different diagnostic criteria.

Tic Disorders: Up to 30% of individuals with OCD also have a lifetime Tic Disorder. A co-morbid Tic Disorder is most common in males with onset of OCD in childhood. These individuals tend to differ from those without a history of Tic Disorders in the themes of their OCD symptoms, co-morbidity, course, and pattern of familial transmission. A triad of OCD, Tic Disorder, and Attention Deficit Hyperactivity Disorder can also be seen in children.

Course and Prognosis

If OCD is untreated, the course is usually chronic, often with waxing and waning symptoms. Some individuals have an episodic course, and a minority of patients have a deteriorating course. Without treatment, remission rates in adults are low (e.g., 20% for those re-evaluated 40 years later); however, up to 40% of individuals with onset of OCD in childhood or adolescence may experience remission by early adulthood.

The pattern of symptoms in adults can be stable over time, but symptoms are much more variable in children. Differences in the content of obsessions and compulsions between children and adults likely reflect content appropriate to different developmental stages (e.g., higher rates of sexual and religious obsessions in adolescents than in children; higher rates of harm obsessions [e.g., fears of catastrophic events, such as death or illness to self or loved ones] in children and adolescents than in adults).

Differential Diagnosis

Several other conditions can appear with obsessive thoughts and therefore need to be considered when making the diagnosis. OCD is also frequently misdiagnosed (see Table 3.1).

Tic Disorder: A tic is a sudden, rapid, recurrent, non-rhythmic motor movement or vocalization (e.g., eye blinking, throat clearing). Tics are typically less complex than compulsions and are not aimed at neutralizing obsessions. Distinguishing between complex tics and compulsions can be difficult. Whereas compulsions are usually preceded by obsessions, tics are often preceded by premonitory sensory urges. Some individuals have symptoms of both OCD and a Tic Disorder, in which case both diagnoses may be warranted.

Stereotypic Movement Disorder (SMD): Stereotypic Movement Disorder (SMD) involves repetitive engagement in motor activities, including head banging, body rocking, self-biting, and hand waving that begin in the early developmental period. Oftentimes these compulsive behaviors are associated with developmental delays although they also occur in young typically developing children. Stereotypic Movement Disorders are differentiated from OCD in that they are fixed, localized, and purposeless (i.e., they are not done in response to an obsessional thought).

Psychotic Disorders: Some individuals with OCD have poor insight or even delusional OCD beliefs. This is not the same as a psychotic disorder or schizophrenia. People with OCD have obsessions and compulsions (distinguishing their condition from delusional disorder) and do not have other features of schizophrenia or schizoaffective disorder (e.g., hallucinations or formal thought disorder). Many people with OCD, however, have been incorrectly diagnosed and treated for psychotic disorders.

Generalized Anxiety Disorder: Recurrent thoughts, avoidant behaviors, and repetitive requests for reassurance can also occur in anxiety disorders. The recurrent thoughts that are present in generalized anxiety disorder (i.e., worries) are usually about real-life concerns, whereas the obsessions of OCD usually do not involve real-life concerns and can include content that is odd, irrational, or of a seemingly magical nature. In addition, compulsions are often present and usually linked to the obsessions.

Specific Phobia: Like individuals with OCD, individuals with specific phobia can have a fear reaction to specific objects or situations (e.g., heights, flying, spiders). In specific phobia, however, the feared object is usually much more circumscribed, and rituals (i.e., compulsions) are not present.

Social Anxiety Disorder: In social anxiety disorder, the feared objects or situations are limited to social interactions, and avoidance or reassurance seeking is focused on reducing this social fear.

Anorexia Nervosa: OCD can be distinguished from anorexia nervosa in that in OCD the obsessions and compulsions are not limited to concerns about weight and food.

Bipolar disorder: Although bipolar disorder appears to be a rare co-morbidity in patients with OCD (2% current rate), when present, it poses a therapeutic dilemma. Specifically, agents (including SRIs) documented to be helpful in the treatment of OCD also have the risk of exacerbating mood symptoms and precipitating mania. Lithium, anti-epileptics, or atypical antipsychotics may therefore be needed to counteract the activating effects of SRIs required to treat OCD. From a drug interaction perspective, SRIs and antipsychotic medications are generally safe to co-prescribe.

Body Dysmorphic Disorder: Body Dysmorphic Disorder, a preoccupation with a slight or imagined defect in appearance, co-occurs with OCD at the rate of approximately 15%. When present, Body Dysmorphic Disorder co-morbidity has been associated with greater depressive symptoms and more illicit drug use. Although Body Dysmorphic Disorder is not associated with more severe OCD, the fact that patients with both disorders have more severe depressive

TABLE 3.1 Frequent Misdiagnoses in Patients with OCD

Misdiagnosis	*Reason for Misdiagnosis*
Depression	Depression often coexists with OCD (25%–30%) and the depression is diagnosed but the OCD missed
Social Phobia or avoidant personality disorder	Because social anxiety is a common consequence of OCD (40%), OCD is often misdiagnosed as Social Phobia or avoidant personality disorder
Agoraphobia	Some patients with OCD are housebound and these patients can be misdiagnosed with agoraphobia
Psychotic disorder	Because the beliefs associated with OCD can be of delusional intensity, some patients are diagnosed with a psychotic disorder
Compulsive sexual behavior or pedophilia	OCD patients who suffer from sexual obsessions will describe intrusive thoughts about sexual activities, sometimes with children. Clinicians unfamiliar with the "taboo" obsessive subtype of OCD will often misdiagnose these patients with sexual addiction or pedophilia
Substance Use Disorder	Chemical dependency in OCD patients is often a response to untreated OCD. Because certain psychoactive substances, such as opiates, may be enticing for individuals with OCD as they may potentially alleviate obsessional symptoms, patients with OCD may develop a Substance Use Disorder. The Substance Use Disorder is then usually diagnosed instead of the underlying OCD
Obsessive Compulsive Personality Disorder	Focusing on the behavior, such as perfectionism or list-making, without assessing whether it is ego-syntonic or dystonic or whether it involves the need for order, symmetry, and arranging may result in misdiagnosis of OCD as OCPD

TABLE 3.1 Continued

Misdiagnosis	*Reason for Misdiagnosis*
Attention Deficit Hyperactivity Disorder	OCD patients with "incompleteness" or "just right" symptoms often display low motivation, repeating rituals, which often resemble procrastination, and difficulties with attention and focus

symptoms and are more likely to use drugs means that treatment strategies need to focus on these related aspects of care.

Monitoring Treatment

Fear about doing exposure therapy may be pronounced in many individuals with OCD. Careful explanation about the gradual process of exposures and the potential benefits of exposure therapy need to be discussed.

Similarly, fear may be present about taking medications. Physicians may need to have frequent visits and discussions regarding medications and their side effects. If the patient has fears about having a psychotic disorder and going "crazy" (not an uncommon obsessive thought), the use of antipsychotic augmentation requires sensitive explanation.

Scales

There are several valid and reliable measures that can be used to monitor change in symptoms during treatment.

Yale-Brown Obsessive Compulsive Scale (YBOCS) is a 10-item clinician-administered scale asking about obsessions and compulsions (e.g., frequency, distress, ability to control) during the past week. General cut-off scores for the YBOCS have been associated with level of OCD severity: 8–15 mild, 16–23 moderate, 24–31 severe, and >32 extreme.

The Obsessive Compulsive Inventory (OCI) is a 42-item scale composed of 7 subscales: Washing, Checking, Doubting, Ordering, Obsessing (i.e., having obsessional thoughts), Hoarding, and Mental Neutralizing. Each item is rated on a 5-point (0–4) scale of symptom distress. Mean scores are calculated for each of the seven subscales and an overall mean "distress" score is calculated. Each score is presented as a mean out of a possible maximum of "4" with lower scores meaning less severe symptoms. A total score of 42 or more, or a mean score of 2.5 or more in any of the subscales, suggests the presence of OCD.

Note: *The OCI is not meant to be diagnostic* but can help the clinician to determine the severity of OCD symptoms.

The Maudsley Obsessive Compulsive Inventory (MOCI) is a 30-question, true/false format, patient-report questionnaire consisting of 4 subscales: checking, washing/cleaning compulsions, slowness, and doubting. Total "true" responses are added to obtain a total score. The scale is split between 15 obsessive questions and 15 compulsive questions but does not cover all such symptoms. As such, the MOCI can assess for certain but not all obsessive or compulsive symptoms.

The Leyton Obsessional Inventory (LOI) is a 69-question, self-report instrument designed to assess for obsessional symptoms and traits. 46 questions are designed to assess for symptoms of OCD and 23 questions target OC personality traits. For each item the patient endorses, he/she completes a 5-point Likert scale showing their level of resistance to that specific symptom or trait as well as a 4-point interference scale measuring the extent to which that symptom or trait interferes with daily activities.

Treatment

Pharmacotherapy

Strong evidence supports the efficacy of pharmacotherapy with serotonin reuptake inhibitors (SRIs) (this includes the tricyclic antidepressant clomipramine as well as the selective serotonin reuptake inhibitors such as paroxetine, fluvoxamine, fluoxetine, citalopram, escitalopram, and sertraline) for children and adults with OCD.

Approximately 40–60% of OCD patients respond to an SRI, and the mean improvement of symptoms is about 20–40%. The probability of full remission of OCD is only about 12%. Relapse rates after medication discontinuation are approximately 90%. Although clomipramine has yielded a larger effect size than the selective SRIs, many patients have trouble tolerating the side effects of clomipramine.

In light of the fact that SRI treatment more often results in partial remission of OCD symptoms compared to complete remission, and changes in psychosocial functioning often lag behind symptom reductions, examining quality of life and long-term functioning of individuals with OCD is critical.

Poor insight is generally considered to be a patient's relative lack of understanding of the degree to which his or her obsessions and compulsions are unreasonable or excessive. Poor insight has been associated with more severe OCD, co-occurring depression, and somatic obsessions. Poor insight OCD patients appear to respond equally well to SRI treatment as those with good insight, provided they are compliant. The addition of an antipsychotic medication does not appear necessary for the treatment of poor insight OCD. OCD patients with poor insight, however, appear to respond less robustly to exposure response prevention therapy.

Indications/Efficacy

Significant evidence supports the efficacy of serotonin reuptake inhibitors (SRIs) and cognitive-behavioral therapy (CBT) (specifically exposure and ritual prevention [ERP]) in reducing OCD symptoms. Clinical practice guidelines recommend that initial treatment be selected based on five factors: (1) nature and severity of patient symptoms, (2) co-morbid psychiatric and medical conditions, (3) past treatment history, (4) current medications, and (5) patient preferences. In addition, level of impairment, concomitant medications, and availability of treatments also need to be considered when selecting treatment strategies.

Clomipramine and the selective SRIs (SSRIs) are effective in reducing OCD symptoms; however, the SSRIs are recommended as the first-line pharmacological treatment for OCD due to a better adverse event profile.

Pharmacological and CBT treatments have documented evidence as effective monotherapies as well as in a combined treatment strategy. The optimal sequence of treatments has not yet been identified, however, the American Psychiatric Association (APA) guidelines recommend ERP monotherapy for individuals who are motivated to cooperate with ERP demands, do not have severe depressive symptoms, or prefer not to take medications.

In the case of patients who find ERP too frightening, SRIs should be started first and then ERP initiated after the medication has reduced the OCD symptoms and perhaps increased the acceptability of ERP to the patient.

SSRI monotherapy is recommended for individuals who are not able to engage in ERP, report a previous response to an SSRI, or prefer medication treatments over CBT. Typical target doses for adult OCD patients are indicated in Table 3.2. For doses in children, see the child-specific chapter. For elderly patients, more cautious dosing is warranted, with low initial starting doses and more gradual titration.

A combination of SSRI treatment and CBT is recommended for individuals who have other co-morbid conditions that could benefit from SSRI treatment (e.g., major depression, generalized anxiety disorder), or those who show an unsatisfactory response to monotherapy. Combined treatment is also recommended for individuals who prefer to take medications for the shortest possible time as there are data from uncontrolled follow-up studies that suggest that CBT may help to prevent or delay relapse when the SSRI is discontinued.

An earlier age at OCD onset and longer duration of OCD were associated with a poorer response to clomipramine and SSRIs.

TABLE 3.2 Target Doses for Medications for OCD in Adults

Serotonin Reuptake Inhibitors	*Target Dose*
Clomipramine	150–250mg/day
Fluoxetine	40–80mg/day
Sertraline	100–200mg/day
Fluvoxamine	200–300mg/day
Paroxetine	40–60mg/day
Citalopram	40mg/day
Escitalopram	20–30mg/day

Greater baseline severity of OCD and co-morbid tics also associated with poorer response to clomipramine and SSRIs in adults. Other possible treatment moderators have been examined such as depression, personality traits, insight, and expressed emotion. There is not consistent evidence that these variables affect treatment outcome.

Initiation/Ongoing Treatment

Baseline investigations are not needed before starting SSRIs. If clomipramine, an SRI, is started, an EKG at baseline is advised. Serum blood levels of clomipramine should be taken to monitor blood levels of clomipramine and desmethylclomipramine to avoid cardiac and CNS toxicity.

If someone responds to an SSRI, a course of treatment should continue for at least one year. Similarly, if depression or anxiety is co-occurring, medication management for at least one year may be necessary.

Before starting CBT, the clinician should make sure the patient knows the intended number of therapy sessions and the need to perform homework assignments. It is generally accepted that 12–16 sessions of CBT is the typical minimum for treating OCD.

Risks/Side Effects

The clinically most common side effects from SRI medications include: nausea, dry mouth, headache, diarrhea, nervousness, agitation or restlessness, reduced sexual desire or difficulty reaching orgasm, inability to maintain an erection (erectile dysfunction), rash, increased sweating, weight gain, drowsiness, or insomnia.

Rarer but serious side effects: arrhythmias are possible with clomipramine and therefore EKGs need to be performed after each dose change or when adding other medications, paying attention to the QTc. In general, clomipramine should be avoided when using concomitant paroxetine, fluoxetine, or fluvoxamine as they may dramatically increase clomipramine blood levels. Seizures have been reported with the use of clomipramine (1%). Citalopram and escitalopram may lengthen QTc at higher doses.

Augmentation of SRIs

For patients who do not adequately respond to SRIs as monotherapy, the next approach involves augmentation of the SRI. Low-dose dopamine antagonists have the most impressive data for their use with SRIs. Three placebo-controlled studies support the use of risperidone for OCD and demonstrated efficacy for aripiprazole, but the use of quetiapine and olanzapine have produced only mixed results.

One study of ondansetron (4mg) augmentation of fluoxetine in 42 adults with OCD found that ondansetron produced significantly greater improvement in OCD symptoms compared to placebo. Similarly, a double-blind, placebo-controlled study of 23 subjects with treatment-resistant OCD found that once-weekly oral morphine showed significant reduction in OCD symptoms compared to placebo. Finally, based on the hypothesis that OCD is associated with an inflammatory process, celecoxib, an NSAID that selectively inhibits prostaglandin synthesis, was added to fluoxetine and compared to placebo in a double-blind study. The combination of celecoxib plus fluoxetine was significantly more effective in reducing OCD symptoms than fluoxetine alone.

Other augmentation strategies, however, while promising in open-label studies, yielded little benefit or mixed results in double-blind, placebo-controlled studies. Trials of lithium, L-triiodothyronine, clonazepam, buspirone, and topiramate all speak against the efficacy of these medications in combination with SRIs for OCD.

Other Monotherapies

For patients who fail to report any improvement from SRIs, or cannot tolerate the side effects of an SRI, the next approach is to consider an alternate monotherapy. Inositol, a dietary supplement that is a precursor of the second messenger phosphatidylinositol has demonstrated superiority to placebo in one double-blind study. Clonazepam has demonstrated mixed results, venlafaxine failed to separate from placebo, and trazodone resulted in no difference from placebo. Although not including a placebo, controlled studies of buspirone versus clomipramine and phenelzine versus clomipramine both demonstrated similar efficacy between the two medications.

Although preliminary studies suggest that several other medications may be beneficial for OCD (for example, glutamate-modulating agents), these agents currently lack double-blind, placebo-controlled data to support their efficacy. Given that previous trials of medication were often successful in open-label studies and not in placebo-controlled studies, these medications require more rigorous testing.

Psychotherapy

The only type of treatment that has been found to be broadly effective for OCD is cognitive behavioral therapy (CBT). The form of CBT that seems to work fairly well for OCD includes exposure and response prevention (ERP): prolonged exposure to obsessional cues and strict prevention of rituals. ERP entails exposure to situations that provoke obsessive anxiety and then abstaining from rituals. Response rates to ERP range from 63% to 90% with an average reduction of 48% of OCD symptoms. Relapse rates after ERP are relatively low but refusal rates are 25% to 30% and drop-out rates are about 28%.

Typically ERP is conducted on a weekly basis, although severity of the disorder may necessitate more frequent sessions. ERP has shown benefit in many different frequency formats and anywhere from 10–16 sessions (usually 90 minute sessions) may be helpful.

Each session begins with a check on homework progress and ends with a new homework/exposure assignment.

Treatment of Common Co-morbid Disorders

Co-morbidities are the norm rather than the exception in people with OCD. Table 3.3 lists treatment guidance for the most common of these.

Clinical Pearls for Obsessive Compulsive Disorder

- SRI therapy is the first-line pharmacotherapy treatment for children and adults with OCD. In many cases it will be necessary to titrate to doses higher than used in the treatment of depression, in order to achieve clinical response.
- Cognitive behavioral therapy, especially exposure and response prevention (ERP) is the first-line psychotherapy intervention for OCD.
- Since treatment response is often only partial, attending to quality of life and long-term functioning is critical.

TABLE 3.3 How to Treat Common Co-morbid Disorders

Co-morbid Disorder	*Treatment Challenge*
Major Depressive Disorder	Responds to some antidepressants which have no proven efficacy in OCD; CBT skills have demonstrated efficacy for depression
Bipolar Disorder	Treatment of OCD with high dose SRIs may precipitate manic episodes; may need mood stabilizer in place before starting SRI
Obsessive Compulsive Personality Disorder	No proven response of OCPD symptoms to SRIs and therefore may confuse understanding of treatment response. ERP focusing on perfectionism, for example, may be beneficial
Body Dysmorphic Disorder	Less robust response to SRIs and higher rates of suicide attempts. CBT/ERP helpful for Body Dysmorphic Disorder
Substance Use Disorders	Certain drugs of abuse may alleviate OCD symptoms; limited benefit from SRIs for Substance Use Disorders. Exposure therapies have questionable efficacy for Substance Use Disorders

- Misdiagnosis is common. OCD is highly co-morbid with major depression, other anxiety disorders, Tic Disorders, hoarding, and Obsessive Compulsive Personality Disorder (OCPD).
- More than one obsession or compulsion is common. Use materials like the Y-BOCS symptom checklist and scoring sheet to help in determining the nature and extent of obsessions and compulsions present.

Key References

- Dold M, Aigner M, Lanzenberger R, Kasper S. Antipsychotic augmentation of serotonin reuptake inhibitors in treatment-resistant obsessive compulsive disorder: a meta-analysis of double-blind, randomized, placebo-controlled trials. Int J Neuropsychopharmacol. 2013 Apr;16(3):557–74.
- Fineberg NA, Gale TM. Evidence-based pharmacotherapy of obsessive compulsive disorder. Int J Neuropsychopharmacol. 2005 Mar;8(1):107–29.
- World Health Organization. www.who.int/healthinfo/statistics/bod_obsessivecompulsive.pdf

4

Hoarding

Clinical Description

Hoarding is the acquisition of and failure to discard a large number of possessions. It involves substantial distress or impairment in the ability to use living areas of the home for their intended purposes. Hoarding is surprisingly common and is potentially seriously disabling. Significant hoarding has recently been shown to occur in 2–5% of the general population.

Prior to DSM-5, hoarding was mentioned in DSM-IV-TR only in the context of Obsessive Compulsive Personality Disorder (OCPD), but the text suggested that serious hoarding behavior should be considered a form of OCD. Its high prevalence and serious consequences, together with research on its distinctiveness from OCD and OCPD, have led researchers to classify it as a distinct disorder in DSM-5 ("Hoarding Disorder").

Diagnosis

The DSM-5 Diagnostic Criteria for Hoarding Disorder require that the person have persistent difficulty discarding possessions, regardless of their actual value, and that the difficulty is due to a perceived need to save the items. In addition, the person is required to have significant distress or psychosocial impairment due to the hoarding. On a practical level, the DSM-5 diagnosis further requires that the hoarding symptoms result in the accumulation of possessions that congest, clutter, and compromise living areas. As with most the DSM-5 disorders, Hoarding Disorder is only an appropriate diagnosis if the symptoms are not due to another medical condition (e.g., brain injury, cerebrovascular disease, Prader-Willi Syndrome) or another psychiatric disorder (e.g., lack of energy or motivation in depression, delusions in a psychotic disorder, or cognitive deficits in dementia).

The DSM-5 diagnosis allows for several specifiers to be added to the diagnosis of Hoarding Disorder. For example, one specifier is "with excessive acquisition" and applies if the person has difficulty discarding possessions and has excessive acquisition of items that are not needed or for which there is no available space.

Another specifier is whether the person has good, fair, or poor insight (i.e., the person recognizes that hoarding is problematic or the person is generally convinced that hoarding is fine despite evidence to the contrary). In the case of a person who is completely convinced that hoarding is not problematic despite evidence to the contrary, they would receive the specifier of "no insight."

The desire to retain objects of value, either sentimental or financial, is a common feeling. With Hoarding Disorder, however, the difficulty discarding possessions seems driven by fears of losing important things. What is considered worthless or worn-out varies considerably from person to person. The nature of items saved by people who hoard indicates that they are not limited to worthless or worn-out things. The most frequently hoarded items include clothes, newspapers, and magazines. Many of these items, especially clothes, are frequently new and never worn. In some cases, the home may be full of new things that have never been removed from their original packaging or have price tags still attached.

The central feature of Hoarding Disorder is the intention to save possessions. The clutter that results is due to purposeful saving and reluctance to discard. Items are saved because they have sentimental significance, for their potential usefulness, or because they have more intrinsic aesthetic value. The nature of emotional attachment is reflected in the reaction to getting rid of a possession. The emotion experienced by people with hoarding when confronted with the prospect of losing one or more items is either anxiety or a feeling of impending grief. Associated with this is the tendency to assign human-like qualities to possessions. Another form of emotional attachment concerns a sense of comfort and security provided by possessions. The thought of getting rid of a possession appears to violate feelings of safety.

The major consequence of hoarding is disorganized clutter, which elicits great concern from family, friends, and even the broader community. The cluttered space is often unusable and unsanitary, and finding important items may be nearly impossible. In some cases, family members keep the living space from being cluttered, and in such cases, the individual can still receive a diagnosis of Hoarding Disorder if there is sufficient distress of other impairment generated by the behavior.

People who hoard experience distress largely due to the consequences of the behavior (for example, conflict with family members over the clutter) and not the thoughts or behaviors themselves. As such, people with hoarding often display limited insight into the consequences of their acts. Research suggests that functioning is impaired in a variety of domains. People are often unable to use living spaces in the home and in severe cases appliances are not functional and utilities such as water and electricity are shut off. Hoarding poses a serious public health burden (for example, fire hazards, infestations) as well as costs to the public in the form of involvement by social service agencies.

Co-morbidity

Obsessive compulsive disorder. Hoarding has historically been considered a subtype or dimension of obsessive compulsive disorder (OCD)—indeed, it is listed as a symptom on the Yale-Brown Obsessive Compulsive Scale (Y-BOCS) check-list. Approximately 20% of individuals with Hoarding Disorder have OCD. Symptoms of incompleteness, "just right" obsessions, and ordering and arranging compulsions have been found to correspond to hoarding among patients with OCD. Individuals with Hoarding Disorder and OCD also share perfectionism, poor memory confidence, and indecisiveness.

Other anxiety disorders. Studies indicate that General Anxiety Disorder (GAD) and Social Phobia are especially common in Hoarding Disorder (25% of patients).

Mood Disorders. Major depression is the most common co-morbid condition in Hoarding Disorder, occurring in around 50% of patients. Individuals with co-morbid depression might display more sadness, anhedonia, and other depressive symptoms. Depressed individuals with hoarding might react to discarding items with a feeling of loss or grief consistent with a sense of loss reported for people with hoarding problems. Behaviorally, fatigue-related avoidance and apathy may dominate the clinical picture, which is likely to interfere with treatment.

Attention Deficit Hyperactivity Disorder. Impaired cognitive function (particularly inattention) is common in hoarding. Approximately 28% of people with Hoarding Disorder meet full diagnostic criteria for Attention Deficit Hyperactivity Disorder (ADHD; inattentive subtype). The attention deficits are hypothesized as one of the information-processing problems underlying Hoarding Disorder. They may report high levels of impulsivity and their efforts to organize and discard items are primarily hampered by distractibility and difficulties with executive functioning.

Compulsive Buying and Kleptomania. Studies have confirmed excessive acquiring in the context of hoarding. Compulsive buying is common, and acquisition of free things tends to be excessive. Stealing is another form of excessive acquisition associated with hoarding. Compulsive buying occurs in approximately 61% of individuals with Hoarding Disorder. The frequency of kleptomania in Hoarding Disorder is fairly common (10%).

Course and Prognosis

Hoarding Disorder is associated with a particularly chronic course and poor prognosis for standard treatments using medication and cognitive behavioral therapy. This may be due to many individuals displaying a striking lack of awareness of the severity of their behavior, often resisting intervention attempts and defensively rationalizing their acquisition and saving.

A growing body of evidence points to the substantial social burden imposed by hoarding. A large sample of individuals with self-identified compulsive hoarding reported a mean 7.0 psychiatric work impairment days per month, equivalent to that reported by participants with bipolar and psychotic disorders. Eight percent reported that they had been evicted or threatened with eviction due to hoarding.

Differential Diagnosis

Several other conditions can lead to clutter in the living space and difficulty discarding possessions.

For example, hoarding behaviors occur in individuals with *Prader-Willi syndrome*, a rare genetic disorder associated with short stature, hyperphagia, insatiability, and food-seeking behavior. Many individuals with Prader-Willi syndrome display hoarding behavior, mostly associated with food, but also non-food items as well.

Hoarding associated with *dementia* appears to stem from significant cognitive deterioration rather than from excessive attachment to objects. The person forgets what they have and perhaps repeatedly buys the same things to excess.

Hoarding has also been described in individuals with *schizophrenia*, but the behavior does not appear motivated by a true attachment to objects. For example, paranoia may make throwing things out difficult due to worries that someone is monitoring their garbage.

Available data suggest that a range of insight can characterize Hoarding Disorder. When severe, the hoarding may appear *delusional*, especially if the items are unsanitary. In the context of hoarding, however, this lack of insight may better be characterized as over-valued ideation which involves beliefs about the value or usefulness of possessions. Many individuals with hoarding recognize the problem with their behavior, but their unreasonable ideas about the value of their possessions make it impossible for them to discard. This may appear to an observer as psychotic, but in reality these beliefs about the value and usefulness of possessions may represent part of the disorder.

Obsessive compulsive disorder is the disorder most closely associated with hoarding, and a significant number of individuals with OCD have hoarding symptoms (25–30%). For example, someone with contamination obsessions may find it difficult to discard items because the items cannot be touched with excessive anxiety.

Individuals with *Major Depressive Disorder, GAD*, and/or *Social Phobia* may find it too difficult to clean their homes and discard items due to lack of energy and hopelessness and inability to go outside of the house. They may therefore end up living in squalor similar to someone with hoarding but these individuals do not keep items due to a desire to save or distress from discarding items.

Monitoring Treatment

Monitoring treatment response in a clinical setting is often difficult with Hoarding Disorder. Given that the symptoms focus on the inability to discard and the over-acquisition of items, one can really only assess improvement by examining the level of clutter in the home. Home visits, therefore, are essential for monitoring treatment outcome. Further monitoring by close friends or family members can be beneficial.

Ambivalence about changing behavior is pronounced in individuals with Hoarding Disorder. Monitoring ambivalence is therefore also important.

Scales

There are several valid and reliable measures that can be used to monitor change in symptoms during treatment:

> Saving Inventory-Revised (SIR). The SIR 3-item is a self-report measure with 3 subscales assessing clutter, difficulty discarding, and excessive acquisition.

Hoarding Rating Scale-Interview (HRS-I: Appendix C). The HRS-I is a 5-item semi-structured interview assessing severity of the different dimensions of hoarding: clutter, difficulty discarding, excessive acquisition, distress, and impairment. Items are rated on a 9-point scale from 0 (none) to 8 (extreme). The HRS-I is administered by the assessor in participant's homes at both pre- and post-treatment.

Clutter Image Rating (CIR). The CIR is a series of nine photographs each of a kitchen, living room, and bedroom with varying levels of clutter. Scores for each room range from 1 (least cluttered) to 9 (most cluttered). Participants select the photograph with the level of clutter that most closely resembles their own in each of eleven possible rooms in their home.

Treatment

Pharmacotherapy

Studies have shown that Hoarding Disorder does not usually respond well to medications. The more severe a person's hoarding is, the less likely they will respond to treatment with a serotonin reuptake inhibitor (SRI) (this includes the tricyclic antidepressant, clomipramine, as well as the selective serotonin reuptake inhibitors such as paroxetine, fluvoxamine, fluoxetine, citalopram, escitalopram, and sertraline). Previous studies have however generally involved OCD patients who had hoarding symptoms and not individuals with Hoarding Disorder as it is currently defined in DSM-5.

Indications/Efficacy

Given the limited efficacy data for medications, the first-line treatment for Hoarding Disorder should be cognitive behavioral therapy (CBT).

If medication is used, the usual approach is to start with SSRIs. Even though hoarding is a statistical predictor of poor response, there are still some individuals with hoarding who do respond to SSRIs.

Medications such as SSRIs may also be beneficial especially for co-occurring depression or anxiety. A stimulant may be useful for co-occurring ADHD.

Initiation/Ongoing Treatment

Baseline investigations are not needed before starting SSRIs. If clomipramine, an SRI, is started, an ECG/EKG at baseline is advised. Serum blood levels of clomipramine should be taken to monitor blood levels of clomipramine and desmethylclomipramine to avoid cardiac and CNS toxicity (where such testing is available). If using high dose citalopram/escitalopram, check the QTc is acceptable via an ECG.

If someone responds to an SSRI, a course of treatment should be for at least one year. Similarly, if depression or anxiety is co-occurring, medication management for at least one year is likely to be indicated.

Before starting CBT, the clinician should make sure the patient knows the intended number of therapy sessions, the need to perform homework assignments, and the need for some home visits.

Risks/Side Effects

The clinically most common side effects from SRI medications include: nausea, dry mouth, headache, diarrhea, nervousness, agitation or restlessness, reduced sexual desire or difficulty reaching orgasm, inability to maintain an erection (erectile dysfunction), rash, increased sweating, weight gain, drowsiness, or insomnia.

Rarer but serious side effects include: arrhythmias are possible with clomipramine and therefore EKGs need to be performed after each dose change or when adding other medications, paying attention to the QTc. In general, clomipramine should be avoided when using concomitant paroxetine, fluoxetine, or fluvoxamine as they may dramatically increase clomipramine blood levels. Seizures have been reported with the use of clomipramine (1%). Citalopram/escitalopram may lengthen the QTc at higher doses.

Psychotherapy

The only type of treatment that has been found to be broadly effective for hoarding is cognitive behavioral therapy (CBT). The form of CBT that seems to work fairly well for hoarding includes the following elements: motivational interviewing, several features of cognitive therapy and behavioral practice, and skills training.

The treatment focuses on three hoarding behaviors: excessive acquisition, difficulty discarding or letting go of possessions, and disorganization and clutter that impairs functioning.

The treatment is designed generally to be undertaken in 26 weekly sessions with some sessions completed in the clients' home. The amount of improvement appears to be related to how much homework clients complete.

The first four sessions focus on education about hoarding and the cognitive behavioral model, including efforts to enhance motivation. Acquisition problems are the topic for sessions 5 and 6. During this portion of the workshop participants attempt non-acquiring trips in which they expose themselves to progressively stronger acquiring triggers in order to learn to tolerate urges to acquire. The following four sessions involve cognitive restructuring exercises and practice in imagined and actual discarding situations. Participants are assigned to complete daily sorting and discarding sessions. The final three sessions address difficult discarding and acquiring issues and prepare participants to continue working on their hoarding after the end of the program.

Sessions each begin with a check on homework progress and end with a new homework assignment.

Treatment Choice and Sequencing of Treatment

Based on the limited data, CBT should be the treatment of choice for Hoarding Disorder. Patients should be started with CBT and medication can be used concomitantly or be started after seeing what progress is made with CBT.

Clinical Pearls for Hoarding

- Individuals with Hoarding Disorder often do not seek treatment due to limited insight and stigma associated with the condition
- Weekly cognitive behavioral therapy is the first-line treatment for hoarding
- Therapy should involve some in-home visits where aspects of motivational interviewing, features of cognitive therapy and behavioral practice, and skills training can be used
- SRI treatments are less effective for hoarding compared to OCD
- Hoarding is highly co-morbid with OCD, major depression, Social Phobia, ADHD, and compulsive buying

Key References

- Mataix-Cols D, Billotti D, Fernández de la Cruz L, Nordsletten AE. The London field trial for hoarding disorder. Psychol Med. 2013 Apr;43(4):837–47.
- Pertusa A, Frost RO, Mataix-Cols D. When hoarding is a symptom of OCD: a case series and implications for DSM-V. Behav Res Ther. 2010 Oct;48(10):1012–20.
- Santana L, Fontenelle JM, Yücel M, Fontenelle LF. Rates and correlates of nonadherence to treatment in obsessive compulsive disorder. J Psychiatr Pract. 2013 Jan;19(1):42–53.

5

Body Dysmorphic Disorder

Clinical Description

Body Dysmorphic Disorder (BDD) is a fairly common condition characterized by preoccupation with a perceived defect in one or more aspect of one's physical appearance. This perception is either completely unrelated to reality or is a gross exaggeration of a minor defect. An equal gender distribution is seen in BDD. Typically, patients have poor insight and their beliefs may be held with delusional intensity, persisting despite evidence to the contrary and reassurance from others. Behaviors or activities to "improve" the defect are common, often occur for several hours each day, and may include excessive grooming, exercise, mirror checking, comparisons with other people, make-up application, and "do it yourself" procedures.

The extent of impairment varies from patient to patient, but social dysfunction is pervasive. Patients often isolate to their home, avoid family and friends, dating, and lose their job or stop working altogether due to the obsession with the perceived defect and belief that they are disgusting or sickening to others. Psychiatric hospitalization is also very common. Suicidal ideation occurs in well over half of BDD patients and nearly a third of patients with BDD seen in clinic have attempted suicide at least once in the past. High levels of stress and significantly impaired overall quality of life are the norm in BDD.

Differentiating Body Dysmorphic Disorder from "Normal" Appearance Concerns

It is important to differentiate normal, everyday appearance concerns from those seen in BDD. Everyday grooming behaviors (such as bathing, wearing clean clothes) and concerns about acne, cold sores, as a few examples, are normal, provided they are not extreme. Many, if not most, people in society have concerns about aspects of their appearance, whether it is their weight, the shape of their nose, muscle mass, hair style, etc. People may go running, lift weights, and in some cases explore plastic surgery. BDD is defined by an excessive concern over an aspect of appearance and a general loss of control/obsessionality over aspects of appearance. The person engages in repetitive behaviors in order to "fix" this defect or mask it. For example, a person with BDD who is concerned about their nose will endorse it as "disgusting" (or the like) and may explore multiple surgeries in an effort to fix their perceived defect. An individual concerned that their arms are not big enough (common for men) will engage in excessive weight lifting, isolate to their home, and wear many layers to cover their arms even though they have been perceived by others to be muscular. Steroid misuse is common.

Diagnosis

The specific BDD criteria for DSM-5 can be summarized as follows:

- Preoccupation with a defect or defects in appearance which other people either cannot see, are very minor, or nonexistent
- Repetitive behaviors or mental rituals accompany the preoccupation and may include checking their appearance in the mirror, excessive exercise, comparing their perceived defect to others, skin picking or hair pulling, or seeking reassurance from others (note: this list is not exhaustive)
- Significant distress or impairment in some aspect of functioning which may include their work or ability to socialize which results from the preoccupation with appearance
- The preoccupation cannot be attributed to an eating disorder

DSM-5 also requires the clinician to specify whether the BDD is with or without *muscle dysmorphia*—the belief that one's body type or build is not muscular enough. This subtype is more common in males.

Insight into the patient's beliefs about their perceived defect(s) or flaw(s) is also important and is noted as a specifier in DSM-5. The clinician should specify whether the patient has good or fair insight (e.g., the BDD beliefs are definitely or probably not true), poor insight (e.g., the BDD beliefs are most likely true), or absent of insight (including delusional beliefs) (e.g., the person firmly believes that the BDD beliefs are true).

While the diagnostic criteria in ICD-10 are similar to those in DSM-5, a notable exception is that ICD-10 requires that patients refuse to accept the advice and reassurance of one or more doctors.

Scales

Scales have been developed to aid the clinician in assessing the severity of BDD symptoms, course of illness, and prior treatments. These scales can also assist the clinician in ruling out other phenomenologically similar disorders such as anorexia nervosa or bulimia nervosa:

The Body Dysmorphic Disorder Questionnaire (BDDQ) is a brief, client-administered scale assessing if patients are concerned that a particular area of their body is unattractive and why they believe this area is unattractive. The client is asked to describe the area(s) of dislike and how much time is spent thinking about these perceived defects on a daily basis. The BDDQ rules out bulimia nervosa and anorexia nervosa by asking whether the main body appearance concern centers on being too fat. It further assesses how this bodily preoccupation affects their daily life in terms of functional impairment and the avoidance of certain activities or people.

The Yale-Brown Obsessive Compulsive Scale (BDD-YBOCS: Appendix C) has been modified for BDD to track severity and change over the course of treatment. The YBOCS is a 12-item scale assessing both urges and thoughts to engage in behavior and actual behavior engagement over the preceding week. The BDD-YBOCS has good inter-rater reliability and validity.

Questions to Ask Patients:

1) Are you concerned with your bodily appearance or feel that an area of your body is particularly unattractive?
2) If yes, ask Eating Disorder questions:
   a. What is the lowest weight you have been in the past year?
   b. Do you restrict your food intake?
   c. If no, then ask "Do you often eat large amounts of food and then purge immediately afterwards?"

If "no" to question #2, further assess for the presence of BDD.

If "yes" to #2, explore Eating Disorder criteria.

Co-morbidity and Sequencing Treatment

Major Depressive Disorder (MDD). Both lifetime and current MDD are extremely common in BDD with lifetime MDD seen in over three-quarters of BDD patients. The same medications used to treat BDD should help with depression. In addition, the skills used in cognitive behavioral therapy can be adapted to address the depression simultaneously with the BDD.

Substance Use Disorders (SUDs). Efforts to self-medicate the often disabling obsessions and anxiety associated with BDD can result in Substance Use Disorder; over one-third of patients with BDD will have such co-morbidities. Some individuals feel that their BDD symptoms may actually be helped by the use of opiates and so this may be a common substance of misuse that patients are reluctant to stop. If the substance use is severe, the person may need detoxification and/or residential treatment prior to initiating therapy for BDD. The initial medication treatment of an SRI for BDD, however, can be started at the same time the person starts treatment for a SUD.

Obsessive Compulsive Disorder (OCD). As part of the putative obsessive compulsive spectrum of disorders, OCD has been found to co-occur in 32% of BDD patients. As in the case of depression, the same medications used to treat BDD should help with OCD and the same focus of cognitive behavioral therapy can be adapted to address the triggers of BDD.

Excoriation (Skin Picking) Disorder (SPD). SPD has been shown to co-occur with BDD in between 26–45% of subjects. Some people with BDD pick to improve appearance, but they may also pick beyond concerns for their appearance. In that case, they would have co-occurring SPD. SRIs have not been beneficial for SPD. Other medications such as naltrexone, *N*-acetylcysteine, or antipsychotics may be helpful for SPD. These medications could be started simultaneously with the SRI for BDD. The basics of cognitive behavioral therapy can be used for both disorders, although if picking is present, elements of habit reversal should be added to the overall therapy approach.

Course and Prognosis

Symptoms of BDD typically begin in early adolescence and follow a chronic course, although reports indicate that symptoms often wax and wane over time. For those who develop BDD prior to the age of 18, suicidal ideation and attempts are more common. Symptoms have been shown to improve significantly through evidence-based treatments.

Differential Diagnosis (or, When Is It Really BDD?)

It is extremely important that BDD not be mistaken for other psychiatric illnesses which often mimic the symptoms seen in BDD.

Misinterpreting BDD for a delusional disorder or schizophrenia, for example, and subsequently treating the patient with atypical antipsychotics will likely result in minimal to no symptom improvement, and could actually do harm to the patient. Likewise, misdiagnosing BDD in someone with psychosis could be disastrous, as risks are likely to be missed and treatments are unlikely to be effective.

Bear in mind the following types of psychiatric or medical conditions in which the clinician may mistake BDD as the primary condition:

- *Eating Disorders.* The BDDQ screens for eating disorders by asking, "Is your main concern with your appearance that you aren't thin enough or that you might become too fat?" Given the obsessive preoccupation with appearance noted in both eating disorders and BDD, ruling out eating disorders is of vital importance. If the individual is solely concerned with weight, an eating disorder would be the proper diagnosis.
- *Agoraphobia.* Patients with BDD often isolate themselves in their home and may be seen as agoraphobic. It is important to address the motivation for remaining housebound or limiting their interactions with the world in order to differentiate other anxiety disorders such as agoraphobia from BDD.
- *Schizophrenia or Delusional Disorder.* Many of the signs and symptoms of BDD mirror the positive and negative symptoms of schizophrenia or delusional disorder. In BDD, however, disorganized behaviors are generally absent and the delusions are typically very specific and isolated.
- *Psychotic depression.* Like eating disorders, the obsessive preoccupation with a perceived defect can, at times, border on being delusional. The person with BDD is convinced that a particular area of the body is grossly unattractive. Significant depressive symptoms may accompany obsessions over bodily defects. Psychotic depression can be associated with somatic delusions (e.g., that a part of the body does not exist or does not function properly).

- *Social anxiety disorder.* Social anxiety disorder is common in BDD and patients with BDD will often isolate themselves from social interaction or become reclusive in their home. Unlike social anxiety disorder, however, BDD is based upon a central preoccupation with defects in appearance and the belief that others will reject or laugh at them due to their physical defect(s).

Treatment

Patients with BDD may seek procedures via plastic surgeons. This is to be firmly discouraged since perceived defects occurring in BDD are either imagined or grossly disproportionate. Furthermore, surgical procedures carry risks and BDD symptoms are unlikely to improve following surgery. In fact, symptoms may well worsen, with concern about scars, or concern shifting to other parts of the body, leading to further surgery-seeking behaviors.

Psychotherapy

The use of Cognitive Behavioral Therapy (CBT) has been shown to be efficacious in reducing the symptoms associated with BDD. As the acronym CBT implies, we recommend the use of a combination of cognitive (e.g., challenging the belief that their appearance is defective and unattractive to others) and behavioral (exposure therapy targeting at decreasing the anxiety associated with either seeing themselves in the mirror or presenting themselves to other people) components. Given that BDD is associated with a variety of behaviors, such as skin picking, excessive mirror checking, and weight lifting or other exercising, addressing the behavioral components of BDD is vital.

Aspects of cognitive restructuring are to be used for BDD patients, including exposure and ritual prevention exercises. Cognitive restructuring should focus on the misinterpretation of their bodily features and embellishment of these perceived defects into negative emotions (feelings of worthlessness, anxiety, depression, etc.) and ritualistic behaviors (picking, weight-lifting, etc.). Mindfulness retraining should be used and include working with the patient to see the "whole body" when looking in the mirror (including standing a reasonable distance from the mirror and not inches away) instead of just the perceived defect, using non-judgmental language when they see themselves (i.e., "my lips are red and soft") and how to interact with others without focusing on comparing his or her (for example) nose with the person with whom they are speaking. In addition, broadening the patients' perceptions of their self-worth is important since patients with BDD often associate the defect with self-worth. Finally, aspects of relapse prevention should be implemented and include replacing BDD-related activities with healthy alternatives which may include hobbies the patient abandoned once the BDD-symptoms took over.

Psychological treatments should ideally be conducted twice each week for the first 4–6 weeks and then weekly thereafter. A total of 4–6 months of sessions lasting 60–90 minutes each have been shown to be efficacious in treating BDD. Continual assessment of mood, BDD symptom severity, and suicidal ideation should coincide with each therapy session.

Pharmacotherapy

There are no medications approved by a regulatory body in any country for the treatment of BDD; however, SSRI treatments have been shown to be effective in treating the symptoms of BDD. Given the efficacy demonstrated by fluoxetine and clomipramine, there is reason to believe that the other SSRIs may be effective for BDD (class effect).

The most robust pharmacotherapy at this time is fluoxetine, although at higher doses than used in depressive or anxiety disorders. We recommend titrating fluoxetine to a dose of at least 60mg/day, depending upon tolerability and efficacy at lower doses.

Should fluoxetine fail or if the patient has already taken an adequate course of the medication, then the tricyclic clomipramine should be started at 25–50mg/day, with dose increasing by 50mg every five days. After reaching 150mg/day, the clinician can wait four weeks to judge effectiveness, and then further increase the dose in steps of 50mg every five days as needed. The average target dose is 100–250mg/day, with usual maximum dose being 250mg/day.

It is important to note that antipsychotic medications have not been helpful for individuals with BDD. BDD patients with delusions should be treated with SRIs, not antipsychotic medications.

Risks/Side Effects

All patients with BDD and co-occurring Major Depressive Disorder or symptoms of depression who are taking antidepressant medications should be alerted to the risk of clinical worsening of depressive symptoms and suicidal ideation which have been linked to the use of these medications. Parents or guardians of children who are prescribed antidepressants, regardless of depression history, should be alerted to this risk. Patients taking clomipramine should also be alerted to the increased risk of seizure associated with taking clomipramine. Other side effects associated with clomipramine include nausea, diarrhea, loss of appetite, dry mouth, increased anxiety, blurred vision, dizziness, constipation, trouble concentrating, insomnia, drowsiness, nightmares, increased sweating, decreased libido, impotence, and difficulties having an orgasm.

Treatment Choice and Sequencing of Treatment

Modular cognitive-behavioral therapy (CBT) or serotonin reuptake inhibitors (SRIs) either alone or in conjunction with one another, are first-line treatments of choice for BDD. If the use of CBT provides inadequate symptom relief or when depressive or anxiety symptoms are present, SRIs should augment CBT treatment. SRIs should still be used for patients with delusional BDD.

Dermatologic Consultation

Many patients with BDD pick relentlessly at a specific area of the body, causing significant excoriation, lesions, and open wounds. As such, dermatologic consultation should occur where significant inflammation or damage of the skin occurs at the site of picking.

Clinical Pearls for Body Dysmorphic Disorder

- Cognitive behavioral therapy and SRIs are the treatments of choice
- Rates of suicide are high in individuals with BDD
- BDD is highly co-morbid with excoriation (Skin Picking) Disorder, OCD, Substance Use Disorders, and major depression

Key References

- Bjornsson AS, Didie ER, Phillips KA. Body dysmorphic disorder. Dialogues Clin Neurosci. 2010;12(2):221–32.
- Phillips KA, Wilhelm S, Koran LM, Didie ER, Fallon BA, Feusner J, Stein DJ. Body dysmorphic disorder: some key issues for DSM-V. Depress Anxiety. 2010 Jun;27(6):573–91.

6

Illness Anxiety Disorder (Hypochondriasis)

Clinical Description

Illness Anxiety Disorder is a new term in the DSM-5, which essentially subsumes the disorder formerly known in DSM-IV as "Hypochondriasis." The core feature of Illness Anxiety Disorder (DSM-5) or Hypochondriasis (ICD-10) is an excessive concern that one has (or is likely to develop) a serious but undiagnosed physical illness. This belief may occur in response to physiological (i.e., normal) bodily sensations or, when occurring in the context of an actual physical illness, the anxiety is grossly disproportionate to the severity of that illness. Affected individuals only experience a transient reduction in anxiety when test results are normal and when clinicians provide reassurance; anxiety later increases once more, leading to further healthcare seeking.

Illness Anxiety Disorder occurs with similar frequency in men and women and can occur at any age. Point prevalence estimates vary from 1–10% in the background population and may be higher in enriched healthcare environments. Left untreated, the condition can become chronic, ingrained, and difficult to manage. Detailed personal history can be useful; in many cases there may be a history of a close relative or friend having a serious medical condition that was overlooked.

Illness Anxiety Disorder results in considerable distress to affected individuals, but critically can also be extremely functionally impairing. The functional impact of Hypochondriasis (e.g., in terms of elevated unemployment and time off work) can be similar to that of serious medical disorders with known organic bases.

Patients often visit different doctors and keep re-presenting themselves to various family doctors and outpatient clinics, which can be very challenging to healthcare professionals who are faced with a dilemma:

1. Investigate further when there is in fact negligible risk of an underlying physical illness, and thereby provide transient relief for the patient and clinician; or
2. Risk the possibility of being perceived as rejecting the patient by recommending against further investigations

Encourage Psychiatric Consultation

The nature of the disorder means that patients often present to family and medical doctors but are avoidant of seeing psychiatrists. Where Illness Anxiety Disorder is suspected, however, every effort should be made to encourage the patient to see a psychiatrist. Rather than telling patients that they should see a psychiatrist because their symptoms have "no physical basis" (which will likely result in the patient refusing to go down this route), useful statements can be:

> "These symptoms are really affecting you and I can understand it's frustrating that we can't find a clear cause. Would you consider seeing a psychiatrist to explore the effects of these problems on your life, and to see if there's anything else we can do to help?"
>
> "Some treatments offered by psychiatrists, such as talk therapy or medication, can help in coming to terms with the effects of medical conditions. This is true even where we haven't identified a clear medical cause. Would you be willing to consider seeing a psychiatrist?"
>
> "There's a lot about the human body that we don't understand. It might be helpful for you to see a psychiatrist to help

come to terms with these uncertainties and frustrations, especially as we haven't identified a clear physical cause for your concerns. Would you consider seeing a psychiatrist?"

Diagnosis

The DSM-5 Diagnostic Criteria for Illness Anxiety Disorder requires that the person is preoccupied with either having or acquiring a major medical disease, that they have somatic symptoms, that high levels of anxiety are present concerning their health and well-being, and that the person displays signs of excessive health-related behaviors (e.g., checking for signs and symptoms of a medical disease) or extreme avoidance (e.g., avoiding healthcare professionals or institutions).

The DSM-5 requires that these symptoms have existed for at least 6 months, although the focus of illness could change during that time (for example, 2 months worrying about cancer and 4 months worrying about HIV/AIDS).

The DSM-5 further requires that these symptoms are not solely attributable to another mental disorder.

The disorder may also receive further specifiers such as *care-seeking type* if medical care is frequently used or *care-avoidant type* if medical care is rarely used.

ICD-10 criteria for Hypochondriasis are similar to those of DSM-5 Illness Anxiety Disorder, with the following two exceptions:

1) There is no minimum time period specified (as compared to the >6 months requirement in DSM-5); and
2) It is made explicit that the preoccupation persists despite appropriate medical investigations and reassurance.

Further, ICD-10 considers Body Dysmorphic Disorder a form of Hypochondriasis, while DSM considers it to be a separate disorder.

Co-morbidity

More than half of patients with Illness Anxiety Disorder will present with co-morbid psychiatric conditions. The most common co-morbidities are:

Depression. Depression is found in up to 33% of people with Illness Anxiety Disorder and a smaller additional proportion will have subsyndromal depression (i.e., dysthymia [20%]). Patients with Illness Anxiety Disorder may develop depressive symptoms following years of frustration and anxiety over their perceived failure of the healthcare system to locate and treat their fictional ailments.

Anxiety Disorders. Illness Anxiety Disorder often co-exists with Generalized Anxiety Disorder (GAD; 25% of patients), Somatization Disorder (20%), and OCD (10%). Patients often report excessive worry associated with Illness Anxiety Disorder. It is important that the clinician screens for the presence of an anxiety disorder and treat it accordingly.

Interestingly, Hypochondriasis is not particularly associated with elevated risk for substance misuse.

Course and Prognosis

Illness Anxiety Disorder can occur at any age but there may be a history of health-related concerns dating back to adolescence upon careful medical history taking. Risk of Hypochondriasis does not appear to be influenced by education levels or income. Very little information is available regarding the longitudinal course of the illness. The few available studies show that over half of people with Illness Anxiety Disorder will experience persisting and functionally impairing symptoms over time without appropriate intervention. While spontaneous resolution of symptoms does occur in a minority of individuals, treatment should be considered for all because spontaneous resolution occurs unpredictably (i.e., no clear predictive factors have yet been identified).

Differential Diagnosis (or, When Is It Really Hypochondriasis?)

Prior to interviewing the patient, it is good practice to review the case records and investigations of the patient to date (if available), to help ensure that medical disorders have not been overlooked and in order to help prepare one's approach towards the patient. Do not rely on statements from other clinicians that the basis of the patient's presentation is clearly "psychiatric" in nature. Keep in mind that some medical conditions can have a psychiatric presentation—e.g., multiple sclerosis and (para)thyroid dysfunction. Having considered this beforehand, the clinician is in a position to provide appropriate firm reassurance and avoid succumbing to requests for unnecessary investigations, which can serve to perpetuate Illness Anxiety Disorder rather than to alleviate it. Even if Illness Anxiety Disorder is confirmed, periodically review the patient's symptoms and presentation in the event that medical conditions have indeed developed.

In addition to considering the possibility of underlying medical disorders, it is important also to differentiate Illness Anxiety Disorder from these other psychiatric conditions:

- *Somatic Symptoms Disorder*. This DSM-5 term encompasses individuals formerly diagnosed with Somatization Disorder. The hallmark of Somatic Symptoms Disorder is excessive focus on a plethora of bodily symptoms (e.g., aches, pains, rumblings) that often change over time; the individual will fixate on talking about these, and their impact on day-to-day life, rather than expressing concern that a specific disorder has been missed. The key to differentiating these conditions lies partly in sensitive exploration of the patient's experiences and whether they have any particular worries about what the cause of the symptoms might be.
- *Chronic Fatigue Disorder*. This is not a psychiatric disorder as such but shares parallels with Somatic Symptoms Disorder above, and can be confused for Illness Anxiety Disorder. Core

features are joint pain, muscle pain, lymph node tenderness, headache, sore throat, poor sleep, general malaise persisting >24 hours after exertion, and subjective memory problems (four or more of these required for diagnosis).

- *Generalized Anxiety Disorder.* People with this condition have excessive anxieties about a variety of events and activities occurring as part of day-to-day life. Examples include pervasive and disproportionate concerns about job responsibilities, health and finances, and the health of family members. The clinician should try to differentiate between patient concerns over their perceived physical health as it relates to having or obtaining an illness versus concerns over work, school, relationships, etc.
- *Social Anxiety Disorder (or Social Phobia).* Individuals fear and avoid situations when they may be exposed to the scrutiny of others (public speaking, being in bars/restaurants, meeting new people). They fear negative evaluation by others. Exposure to given situations nearly always provokes anxiety and/or avoidance. The underlying concerns relate to external cues rather than internal somatic experiences.
- *Panic Disorder.* The distinguishing feature of Panic Disorder as compared to Illness Anxiety Disorder is the occurrence of discrete periods (abrupt onset, peaking within 10 minutes) of intense fear and/or discomfort and physiological sensations (e.g., tachycardia, shallow rapid breathing leading, sweating, dizziness). These discrete events may at the time be perceived to be a medically significant event (e.g., a heart attack). After one or more panic episodes, the patient tends to worry about panic attacks recurring and associated embarrassment plus loss of control, rather than seeking medical attention because they believe specific medical disorders have been missed.
- *Body Dysmorphic Disorder (BDD).* Here, the individual is preoccupied with the belief that he or she has one or more defects in their outward physical appearance rather than having a labeled medical condition. In Illness Anxiety Disorder, sufferers are worried that an internal disorder is not "noticeable"

to others (i.e., is being overlooked), while in BDD, subjects believe their perceived deficits are very noticeable to others and consequently attempt to avoid exposure. Excessive checking and reassurance seeking nonetheless commonly occur in both conditions.

- *Obsessive Compulsive Disorder (OCD).* There are many parallels between Illness Anxiety Disorder and OCD: both involve recurrent intrusive thoughts and compulsions undertaken in a rigid way and/or in response to these thoughts. A diagnosis of OCD is more appropriate when the nature of obsessions and compulsions generalize to other domains besides the belief that there is an unrecognized serious medical disorder. It can be helpful to use the Yale-Brown Obsessive Compulsive Scale (YBOCS) symptom checklist to help detect the presence of symptom types more likely to be due to OCD (see OCD chapter).

Scales

The Whiteley Index is a 14-item self-complete questionnaire, which poses a variety of questions in binary form ("no" or "yes"). A total score of 5 or more on the Whiteley Index is strongly suggestive of Hypochondriasis. This is quite a useful instrument for quick screening.

The Hypochondriasis Yale-Brown Obsessive Compulsive Scale Modified (H-YBOCS-M: Appendix C) is a clinician-administered scale and is recommended for tracking response to treatment. It considers illness thoughts / worries, illness-related behaviors, and illness-related unhealthy avoidance (i.e., three domains rather than the two in the original YBOCS used for OCD). Within each domain there are six questions, each scoring 0–4 with higher scores indicating greater severity. This generates a total score (range 0–72) and three sub-scale scores (each range 0–24). There is an additional item in the H-YBOCS-M quantifying insight (0–4) though this is not utilized in the summary scores. As a rough guide, total Hypochondriasis severity scores can be categorized as: no Hypochondriasis (0), minimal Hypochondriasis (1–12), moderate Hypochondriasis (13–41), severe Hypochondriasis (42–56), and extreme Hypochondriasis (57–72). We recommend that treatment response be defined as a 35% or greater reduction in total severity score as this has been shown to be an indicator of treatment response in clinical research trials of similar conditions.

Treatment

Having ruled out (as far as practically possible) underlying medical conditions and confirmed the probable diagnosis of Illness Anxiety Disorder, attention should turn to treatment options.

Pharmacotherapy

Few pharmacological trials for the treatment of Illness Anxiety Disorder have been conducted. Some evidence, mostly from open-label studies (meaning studies where all patients received the active medication without some sort of control group), supports the use of SSRIs in Hypochondriasis. Where SSRIs are used, we advise using dosing regimens akin to those found to be effective for OCD (see OCD chapter). This recommendation is based on clinical similarities between these two conditions.

In a double-blind study conducted in Hypochondriasis, 16-week treatment with the SSRI paroxetine was superior to placebo for those who completed the trial but failed to demonstrate efficacy for those who discontinued early. The dosing regimen for paroxetine was 10mg/day in week 1, 20mg/day in week 2, with subsequent dosing increments of up to 20mg/day for each week of treatment, to a maximum of 60mg/day. Similar positive results were found in another double-blind placebo-controlled study using fluoxetine. The dosing regimen for fluoxetine was 20mg/day increasing by 20mg/day every two weeks as needed and tolerated, up to a maximum of 80mg/day.

When patients with Hypochondriasis were treated with 12-week SSRI (fluoxetine/fluvoxamine) and followed up later (mean ~9 years later), 40% still met criteria for Hypochondriasis. Interval treatment with an SSRI for at least one month was associated with greater rates of remission at follow-up (80% versus 40% remission rates).

Psychotherapy

In a meta-analysis, treatment of Hypochondriasis with several types of psychotherapy was associated with significant benefits compared to waiting list control (i.e., no treatment): cognitive therapy, behavioral therapy, cognitive behavioral therapy, and behavioral stress management. Total therapist time ranged from 4–19 hours, and effect sizes correlated significantly with total therapist time (more time = greater benefits). Psychoeducation alone was not beneficial compared to wait-list control.

Treatment Choice and Sequencing of Treatment

It is important to seize opportunities to identify and aggressively treat Illness Anxiety Disorder for several reasons. The condition seldom remits without treatment and is associated with functional outcomes akin to that seen in severe medical conditions with known organic bases. Without treatment, patients are likely to "doctor shop" and undergo many unnecessary and expensive medical examinations and investigations, which only serve to perpetuate the illness. Due to the likelihood of the patient seeking care from more than one doctor, psychiatrists and practitioners in other fields (e.g., family doctors) should work together to treat the patient in a unified way, ideally with joint patient meetings where possible.

Treatment of Choice

We recommend concomitant treatment with psychological intervention (e.g., cognitive behavioral therapy, ideally total therapist contact >10 hours) and an SSRI prescribed at a dose akin to those used in Obsessive Compulsive Disorder.

In addition, we recommend the following:

- Offer regularly scheduled follow-up visits. This can be useful in your efforts to reduce escalation, patient frustration, and "doctor shopping" and will encourage the development of a therapeutic alliance over time and facilitate monitoring of treatment response.
- Avoid changing the frequency and length of sessions as a function of symptom number or severity. This can lead to reinforcement of maladaptive healthcare seeking behaviors.
- Acknowledge the seriousness of the patient's symptoms and the impact they are having on their life, however, the clinician should avoid giving categorical assurances that symptoms will improve or particular treatments will work.
- The onset of new symptoms or endorsement of symptoms should prompt the clinician to consider whether an underlying medical disorder could be present. They should not be ignored.
- Patients should be dissuaded from inappropriate visits to the emergency room.

Clinical Pearls for Illness Anxiety Disorder (Hypochondriasis)

- First-line treatment is psychological intervention (cognitive therapy / behavioral therapy, and stress management)
- Strongly consider also starting an SSRI, and titrating to doses used for OCD
- Regular but short scheduled appointments with a trusted clinician can help avert crises and inappropriate presentations to the emergency room
- Highly co-morbid with depression and anxiety disorders (GAD, Somatization Disorder, and OCD)

- Keep an open mind about the possibility of any underlying medical conditions but avoid feeding into patient anxiety and excessive medical investigations

Key References

- Abramowitz JS, Braddock AE. Hypochondriasis: conceptualization, treatment, and relationship to obsessive compulsive disorder. Psychiatr Clin North Am. 2006 Jun;29(2):503–19.
- Thomson AB, Page LA. Psychotherapies for hypochondriasis. Cochrane Database Syst Rev. 2007 Oct 17;(4):CD006520.

7

Trichotillomania (Hair Pulling Disorder)

Clinical Description

Trichotillomania, also known as Hair Pulling Disorder, is characterized by the repetitive pulling out of one's hair leading to hair loss and functional impairment. In order to qualify for a diagnosis, the hair loss must not be due to another psychiatric or medical condition. The most common sites pulled include the scalp, eyebrows, and eyelashes although pulling from other areas of the body is frequent. Pulling from multiple sites is common and pulling episodes can last from a few minutes to several hours.

Onset of hair pulling is generally in late childhood or early adolescence although onset of pulling behaviors can occur at any age. In adults, Trichotillomania has a large female preponderance, however in childhood, the sex distribution has been found to be equal. Trichotillomania is associated with reduced self-esteem and avoidance of social situations due to shame and embarrassment from the pulling and its consequences—it has a negative impact on quality of life. Patients often perceive Trichotillomania as nothing more than a "bad habit" rather than being a recognized psychiatric condition, and the majority have never sought treatment or discussed their pulling behaviors with health care professionals. Indeed, patients commonly have never disclosed their symptoms to anyone. Avoidance of activities, such as getting haircuts, swimming, being outside on a windy day, sporting activities, dating, or going out in public more than necessary are quite common. Many individuals conceal areas in which they have pulled hair with hats, scarves, bandanas, make-up or by wearing concealing clothing.

Individuals with Trichotillomania often report significant urges or a "drive" to pull their hair. Triggers to pull vary from person to person. Cues prompting pulling episodes may include stress, boredom, "downtime," fatigue, or driving. Many patients report not being fully aware of their pulling behaviors, also referred to as "automatic" pulling and comprise a more habitual form of the disorder. Conversely, "focused" pulling generally occurs when the patient sees or feels a hair that is "not right" (e.g., the hair may feel coarse, fine, sharp, rough, oily, or dry, or appear too dark, curly, gray, or "out of place"). Most patients pull with varying degrees of focused and automatic pulling.

Trichotillomania can result in unwanted medical consequences. Pulling of hair can lead to skin damage if sharp instruments, such as tweezers or scissors, are used to pull the hairs. Over 20% of patients eat hair after pulling it out (trichophagia), which can result in gastrointestinal obstruction and the formation of intestinal hair-balls (trichobezoars) requiring surgical intervention.

Diagnosis of Trichotillomania

The criteria for Trichotillomania in DSM-5 can be summarized as follows:

- Pulling of hair which results in hair loss
- The person endorses trying to either stop pulling or cut down on pulling
- The patient experiences distress as a result of pulling or some aspect of social, work, or other area of functioning is impaired
- Another medical condition is not responsible for the pulling
- Another mental health condition (such as pulling to improve one's appearance or a perceived defect as seen in Body Dysmorphic Disorder) is not the main prompt for pulling

[Note: there are two key differences between DSM-5 and its predecessor in DSM-IV-TR, in terms of diagnostic criteria for Trichotillomania. Firstly, in DSM-IV-TR, hair loss needed to be "noticeable" for a diagnosis; for DSM-5, hair loss need not be noticeable. This diagnostic change recognizes that hair loss is often masked by patients, e.g., by using wigs or cosmetics. Secondly, DSM-5 does not require pleasure, gratification, or relief resulting from pulling, while DSM-IV-TR did. This diagnostic change stems from the recognition that at least 10% of people with hair pulling do not endorse these feelings, which in any event are quite subjective.]

The *ICD-10* classifies Trichotillomania (or hair plucking or pulling) as an impulse disorder. The ICD criteria for a diagnosis of Trichotillomania include:

1) Excessive pulling of one's own hair resulting in noticeable hair-loss;
2) Hair-pulling is usually preceded by mounting tension;
3) Pulling is followed by a sense of relief or gratification

ICD-10, like the DSM system, denotes that a diagnosis of Trichotillomania should not be made if there is a pre-existing inflammation of the skin due to other causes. ICD-10 also highlights the need to exclude stereotyped movement disorder and hair pulling undertaken in response to delusions or hallucinations.

Scales

Several scales have been developed in order to aid the clinician in assessing the severity of hair pulling symptoms and treatment response:

National Institute of Mental Health Trichotillomania Symptom Severity Scale (NIMH-TSS) is a 6-item, clinician-administered scale that rates hair pulling symptoms during the past week (although only four items are scored and two of these questions are directly related to the time spent engaged in pulling). The items assess pulling frequency (both on the previous day and during the past week), urge intensity, urge resistance, subjective distress, and interference with daily activities. The scale takes less than 5 minutes to administer.

Massachusetts General Hospital Hair Pulling Scale (MGH-HPS: Appendix C) is a 7-item, self-report scale that rates urges to pull hair, actual amount of pulling, perceived control over behavior, and distress associated with hair pulling over the past seven days. Analysis of the MGH-HPS has demonstrated two separate factors with acceptable reliability for both "severity" and "resistance and control." Unlike the NIMH-TSS scale, the MGH-HPS scores for urges to engage in the pulling behavior (the first three questions) along with actual pulling behavior, and therefore may more comprehensively capture the pathology. The scale takes approximately 5 minutes to complete.

Differential Diagnosis (or, When Is It Really Hair Pulling Disorder?)

Bear in mind the following types of psychiatric or medical conditions in which the clinician may mistake Trichotillomania as the primary condition:

- *Alopecia areata*: A relatively common autoimmune disease resulting in the loss of hair affecting approximately 2% of the population. It typically causes smooth, roundish patches of hair loss. The disease course is widely variable and highly unpredictable.

  Ask: "Have you been diagnosed with alopecia at any time in your life? Do you find that your hair falls out naturally?" Be on guard for organic causes of hair loss—especially where patients are denying that they pull out their hair. Seek a dermatological consultation where there is any suspicion of alopecia areata.
- *Stimulant use*: It is not uncommon for individuals who use stimulants, either illicit ones or by prescription, to report

worsening of their hair pulling in response to skin sensations resulting from drug use. It may be unclear whether someone has Trichotillomania caused by stimulant use, but is fairly common that stimulant use exacerbates the pulling. To examine the severity of the pulling, however, the clinician should ask about any use of stimulants.

Ask: "Do you use any stimulants (note: give examples if the patient is unclear what is meant by 'stimulants')? If yes, have you noticed if using these substances makes the hair pulling worse?"

- *Body Dysmorphic Disorder (BDD)*: BDD is characterized by obsessions about and preoccupation with a perceived defect of one's physical appearance. In BDD, individuals may pull hair with the aim of correcting a perceived defect of their appearance (e.g., "I know that my arms are too hairy and disgusting to people").

  Ask: "Do you pull out your hair to improve your looks?" If yes, then explore rest of BDD criteria.
- *Excoriation (Skin Picking) Disorder*: While Trichotillomania and Skin Picking Disorder often co-occur, it is important from a treatment standpoint to determine the primary condition since treatments that work for skin picking (such as SSRIs) have shown limited efficacy in Trichotillomania and vice versa. Many patients pick at their skin in order to get to a hair root and this should be diagnosed as Trichotillomania and not Skin Picking Disorder. If the patient picks with the secondary purpose of, for example, fixing a perceived blemish on the skin or a "bump," Skin Picking Disorder is the proper diagnosis.

  Ask: "Do you pick at your skin in order to get to ingrown hairs or the root of hairs?"

The differentiation of Trichotillomania from these other dermatological and psychiatric conditions can be aided by using tools such as client-administered Body Dysmorphic Disorder Questionnaire (BDDQ), referral to a dermatological specialist, and assessing for the use of illicit substances during initial patient presentation.

Hair loss itself, not due to pulling out of one's hair, has a multitude of potential causes. When considering differential diagnoses for Trichotillomania, especially where the individual denies hair pulling, the following possibilities should be considered (along with alopecia areata):

- Hair loss secondary to certain medical conditions (thyroid dysfunction or other endocrine disturbance, scalp infections, e.g., ringworm, other skin conditions. e.g., lichen planus, eczema, seborrheic dermatitis), or suspected hormonal influences (pregnancy, childbirth, discontinuation of birth control pills, and onset of menopause).
- Vitamin/nutritional factors (low iron [check "ferritin"] has been associated with hair loss, and responds to iron treatment; there is only limited evidence that zinc deficiency causes hair loss, despite this being a popular belief, but zinc supplements may help some people). Paradoxically, excessive use of nutritional supplements may trigger hair loss in some otherwise healthy people.
- Medication-induced hair loss (certain agents used to treat these conditions are particularly implicated: arthritis, cancer [e.g., chemotherapy], cardiovascular disease). Make a list of current medications and check product information characteristics as to whether hair loss is a known side effect. If medication is a possible cause, this should be discussed with the patient.
- Hereditary hair loss (male-pattern baldness and female-pattern baldness): there will often be a family history and similar temporal pattern in relatives. Onset can occur from puberty and may be influenced by hormonal factors.
- Loss of hair due to traction: e.g., hair that is tightly drawn up into a bobble on a recurrent basis.
- Physical or emotional shock/insult: there are case reports of general hair thinning in the months following a significant physical or emotional shock. This can include extreme weight

loss from any cause and malnourishment such as seen in anorexia nervosa.

Co-morbidity and Sequencing Treatment

Co-morbid psychiatric conditions, especially depression and/or anxiety (lifetime histories of which are seen in over 50% of patients) are extremely common in Trichotillomania, and should always be screened for. Clinicians should start by ruling out dermatological conditions such as alopecia areata and psychiatric issues such as substance (especially amphetamine and cocaine) abuse. Hair loss due to dermatological conditions would negate a Trichotillomania diagnosis, while use of such illicit substances can worsen hair pulling and contribute towards the persistence of symptoms.

Major Depressive Disorder (MDD). Lifetime and current MDD are common in Trichotillomania and occur in between 29–52% of patients. The use of medications indicated for depression, including SRIs, should be considered as adjunctive to those indicated for Trichotillomania. If suicidality is present in the patient, however, it should be addressed first prior to the initiation of treatment for Trichotillomania.

Obsessive Compulsive Disorder (OCD). OCD has been found to co-occur in over 26% of patients with Trichotillomania. If OCD is present, it should be treated first, prior to the treatment of Trichotillomania. This is because hair pulling can occur as a symptom of OCD, and may well improve as OCD improves if this is the case. There is also some evidence that SRI treatment with clomipramine is efficacious in the treatment of stand-alone Trichotillomania. Aspects of habit reversal therapy and cognitive behavior therapy can be adapted to address the triggers associated with Trichotillomania.

Excoriation (Skin Picking) Disorder. Skin picking has been shown to co-occur with Trichotillomania in over 36% of patients. Given their high rate of co-occurrence, a dual-diagnosis with Trichotillomania is often warranted. Different therapeutic strategies have been shown to work in Trichotillomania and Skin Picking Disorder. For example, while SSRIs have been shown to be useful in Skin Picking Disorder, they do not appear to be useful for the majority of Trichotillomania patients. Likewise, *n*-acetylcysteine has been shown to be helpful in adults with Trichotillomania but questions remain about its efficacy in Skin Picking Disorder (with the exception of case reports).

Course and Prognosis

There is considerable variability in the onset and time course of Trichotillomania. The majority of patients report onset between the ages of 8 and 15 years old. Individuals with Trichotillomania are likely to present first with other psychiatric symptoms, including depression and/or anxiety as they may be unaware that Trichotillomania is a recognized and treatable psychiatric condition. Patients are often ashamed of their hair pulling and secretive about it. Even if they have told other people about the habit (e.g., a loved one or friend), this may have been met with dismissiveness or even overt criticism, feeding into help-avoidance and shamefulness. Patients may perceive their pulling as nothing more than a bad habit. As such, it is extremely important to engage with the patient and provide reassurance that many people experience similar symptoms. Like adults with Trichotillomania, children with Trichotillomania are unlikely to self-report their pulling behavior without prompting.

While young children (<5 years old) with Trichotillomania may get better without sequelae, most older children report a chronic course continuing into adulthood with periods of waxing and waning of symptoms.

Adults with Hair Pulling Disorder show functional impairment and lower quality of life, while the impact of childhood symptoms is less well studied. With treatment, however, quality of life, mood, and anxiety symptoms, which may have been impaired prior to treatment, have all been shown to improve with Trichotillomania symptom improvement although positive changes in these aspects of functioning may take a longer time to occur.

Treatment

Pharmacotherapy

There are no labeled medications for the treatment of Trichotillomania; however, a multitude of studies have been conducted examining the safety and efficacy of different pharmacological interventions. Pharmacotherapies which have indicated efficacious outcomes in Trichotillomania include *n*-acetylcysteine (NAC), clomipramine, olanzapine, and dronabinol although each of these treatments has been shown to be efficacious in relatively small samples of clinical trial patients.

The most robust pharmacotherapy at this time is the glutamatergic agent *n*-acetylcysteine (NAC) for adults with Trichotillomania. Adult patients should start treatment at 600mg twice/day for one week, then 1200mg twice/day for up to four weeks, and then 1800mg upon awakening and 1200mg about 10 hours later per day.

An alternative medication for Trichotillomania is the serotonin tricyclic clomipramine, which should be started at 25–50mg/day, with dose increasing by 50mg every five days. After reaching 150mg/day, the clinician can wait four weeks to judge effectiveness, and then further increase the dose in steps of 50mg every five days as-needed. The average target dose is 100–250mg/day, with usual maximum dose being 250mg/day.

Dronabinol, a cannabinoid antagonist and antiemetic, is a synthetic derivative of THC (the active ingredient in cannabis), and may reduce the excitotoxic damage caused by glutamate release in the striatum, offering promise in reducing pulling behaviors seen in Trichotillomania. Dronabinol is a Schedule III controlled substance in the United States and its availability and legal status are likely to differ as a function of world geographical location. Patients should be started on 2.5mg/day for 2 weeks, increasing to 5mg/day for 2 weeks, then 10mg/day for 2 weeks, and finally titrated to a maximum dose of 15mg/day thereafter depending on clinical efficacy and patient tolerability.

Olanzapine can be used, starting at 2.5mg/day for 2 weeks, then increased to 5mg/day for 2 weeks, then 10mg/day for two weeks, and finally a maximum dose of 20mg/day depending on clinical response and tolerability. Given the side effect profile of olanzapine and other antipsychotics, we recommend that these medications only be considered for patients who have failed to respond adequately to NAC or clomipramine treatment in the first instance.

Psychotherapy is considered the treatment of choice for children and adolescents.

Indications/Efficacy

We recommend psychotherapy, specifically habit reversal therapy (HRT), if available (see below) rather than pharmacotherapy as first-line treatment for Trichotillomania, except for adults with moderate-severe illness for whom medication plus therapy is indicated. Adjunctive pharmacotherapy should be considered on a case-by-case basis.

Initiation/Ongoing Treatment

Baseline investigations are generally unnecessary for NAC, in the absence of systemic disease.

For clomipramine, it is best practice to undertake a baseline EKG (ECG). Baseline investigations prior to initiation of antipsychotic medication should include an EKG (ECG), fasting lipid levels and glucose, liver function tests, urea and electrolytes, full blood count, and prolactin; pulse and blood pressure should be recorded along with body mass index and waist circumference. These should be repeated at 6 months, then at 1 year, then annually thereafter (unless there are specific concerns).

Before starting psychotherapy, the clinician should make sure the patient (and family, in the case of children) knows the intended number of therapy sessions, and the need to perform homework assignments.

Risks/Side Effects

The clinically most common side effects from NAC include nausea, indigestion, headache and abdominal pain although it is generally well tolerated. Contraindications include current asthma and current pregnancy/lactation as the effects of NAC on fetal development have not been assessed.

Patients taking clomipramine should also be alerted to the increased risk of seizure associated with taking this medication. Other side effects associated with clomipramine include nausea, diarrhea, loss of appetite, dry mouth, increased anxiety, blurred vision, dizziness, constipation, trouble concentrating, insomnia, drowsiness, nightmares, increased sweating, decreased libido, impotence, and difficulties having an orgasm. Where available, plasma levels of clomipramine (and its metabolite desmethylclomipramine) should be recorded (draw levels 12 hours after last dose and after 7–14 days on the same dose). This can be useful to monitor for high levels that would predispose towards toxicity. Some studies suggest that plasma levels of 100–250ng/mL for clomipramine and 230–550ng/mL for the major metabolite are generally likely to be effective, but these recommendations stem from limited data.

The most commonly reported adverse events from antipsychotic medications include sedation, weight gain, elevated lipids/glucose, and constipation. Rarer but serious side effects of antipsychotics include extra-pyramidal side effects (including acute dystonic reactions), neuroleptic malignant syndrome (NMS), drug-induced Parkinsonism, dry mouth, blurred vision, elevated prolactin (which can lead to sexual dysfunction in men and women), urinary retention, and clinically significant EKG (ECG) changes.

All patients with Trichotillomania and co-occurring Major Depressive Disorder or symptoms of depression who are taking antidepressant medications should be alerted to the risk of clinical worsening of depressive symptoms and suicidal ideation which have been linked to the use of these medications. Parents or guardians of children who are prescribed antidepressants, regardless of depression history, should be alerted to this risk.

The most clinically significant side effects seen with cannabinoid antagonists such as dronabinol include nausea and psychomotor agitation and retardation. As such, extreme caution should be exercised in operating machinery and motor vehicles.

Psychotherapy

Various components of Cognitive Behavioral Therapy (CBT) are the most widely recognized and efficacious treatments for Trichotillomania. These are some of the techniques that have been shown to be effective in reducing hair pulling symptoms for adults with Trichotillomania.

Habit Reversal Therapy (HRT) is relatively well established in the treatment of Trichotillomania, with large effect size versus control conditions. HRT is a first-line treatment and focuses on awareness training (encouraging awareness of situations that can precede pulling episodes); relaxation training (since anxiety and stress are commonly reported triggers for hair pulling episodes); competing response training (encouraging unwanted pulling behaviors to be replaced with a less conspicuous action—e.g., clenching fists or squeezing a stress ball antagonistic to the pulling action); motivation procedures (designed to improve how acceptable HRT is to patients and their families); and generalization training (rehearsing trigger situations and the sequence of starting the pulling episode, quelling it, and undertaking a competing response). There is evidence that a short course of HRT can be as effective as a more protracted course of therapy and that the benefits extend beyond the end of the treatment.

Stress reduction training, in conjunction with habit reversal techniques, is also beneficial in helping patients to reduce pulling and deal with emotion regulation difficulties. Depending on the triggers of the patient, learning how to reduce stress may alleviate some of the intensity of pulling urges and behavior. For example, if the patient reports that high levels of work stress generally trigger a pulling episode in the car on the way home from the office, the clinician can suggest ideas to manage the stress without pulling (such as going for a vigorous walk immediately after work prior to getting in the car).

Cognitive Restructuring

Cognitive restructuring is the process of evaluating, challenging, and changing maladaptive core beliefs that often perpetuate a problem. Since many individuals with Trichotillomania report pulling to reduce a negative thought or mood, cognitive restructuring can help by identifying and changing irrational or negative beliefs which lead to pulling behaviors. Cognitive restructuring involves two steps, the first of which is to identify the thought(s) or belief(s) that prompt a negative thought or emotion. Second, the therapist helps the patient to critically evaluate those thoughts or emotions for accuracy and usefulness. The therapist can then help the patient to replace any inaccurate or irrational thoughts with ones that are more accurate and useful to the patient.

Dialectical Behavior Therapy-Enhanced Habit Reversal Therapy

Mindfulness training techniques have been shown to be efficacious as conjunctive to an acceptance-based treatment components and *Dialectical Behavior Therapy (DBT)*. The therapy consists of mindfulness training (e.g., patients are taught to experience urges or negative emotions as they occur in the present moment and learn to allow them to pass without pulling), teaching patients skills to regulate negative emotions without pulling, and building a distress tolerance (e.g., tolerating urges or stressful events without pulling).

Acceptance and Commitment Therapy (ACT) is a subsidiary component of HRT in which patients are asked to experience urges to pull and accept the urge without acting on it. The negative emotions involved with pulling are also engaged but not acted upon. The idea is that understanding, feeling, and experiencing the fact that the individual does not have to respond to an urge or emotion can help the patient to feel more in control of his or her pulling.

Online Therapy. Online therapeutic tools have also been developed by expert clinicians with a substantial amount of experience treating Trichotillomania, including at www.stoppulling.com. The behavioral therapy offered online seeks to help the patient to identify situations or triggers prompting hair pulling and subsequently strategize ways in which the patient can address and change those behaviors. Online therapy has been reported as particularly useful for individuals living in rural communities, those with a hectic schedule, or for those who prefer to engage in therapy without leaving their home (due to, for example, embarrassment or shame from bald patches where pulling has occurred).

Treatment Choice and Sequencing of Treatment

Cognitive behavioral therapy (specifically components of HRT or ACT) should be started as first-line treatment for Trichotillomania where treatment is indicated. NAC should be considered as adjunctive therapy to CBT or prescribed as mono-therapy in cases where psychotherapy by a trained therapist is unavailable or unrealistic given geographical constraints of the patient or an inability of the patient to make regular appointments. For patients with co-occurring depressive or anxiety disorders, clomipramine combined with CBT may provide lessening of both Trichotillomania and depressive/anxiety symptoms, however, careful monitoring for safety and tolerability are of the utmost importance. Dronabinol is promising as a treatment for Trichotillomania but its availability is limited; it is a controlled substance in many geographical domains and is completely unavailable in others. Online therapy has been shown to be effective in reducing the symptoms of Trichotillomania but is not a replacement for in-person behavior therapy.

Consultation with Other Disciplines

Dermatologic consultation should occur where significant inflammation of the skin occurs at the site of pulling, or where there is diagnostic uncertainty as to the cause of hair loss. Consultation with colleagues can be helpful when an individual denies deliberate hair pulling and to help rule out medical causes for hair loss. For patients who repetitively bite their hair, run in between their teeth, or chew on their hair, dental consultation should also be encouraged.

Clinical Pearls for Trichotillomania

- Habit Reversal Therapy or *n*-acetylcysteine (as monotherapies or combined) are the treatments of choice
- SSRI not clinically useful for people with stand-alone Trichotillomania
- Highly co-morbid with excoriation (Skin Picking) Disorder, OCD, and major depression
- Hair pulling symptoms may have origins in dermatologic (alopecia areata) or psychiatric (illicit substance use [methamphetamine or cocaine], Body Dysmorphic Disorder) conditions which must be ruled out

Key References

- Chamberlain SR, Odlaug BL, Boulougouris V, Fineberg NA, Grant JE. Trichotillomania: neurobiology and treatment. Neurosci Biobehav Rev. 2009 Jun;33(6):831–42.
- Hoppe L, Ipser JC, Fineberg N, Chamberlain S, Stein DJ. Pharmacotherapy for trichotillomania. Cochrane Database of Systematic Reviews 2009, Issue 1. Art. No.: CD007662.
- Sarah HM, Hana FZ, Hilary ED, Martin EF. Habit reversal training in trichotillomania: guide for the clinician. Expert Rev Neurother. 2013 Sep;13(9):1069–77.

8

Excoriation (Skin Picking) Disorder

Clinical Description

Excoriation Disorder, also known as Skin Picking Disorder, Pathological Skin Picking, neurotic/psychogenic excoriation, and Dermatillomania, is a relatively common body-focused repetitive behavior (BFRB) characterized by compulsive picking of skin causing tissue damage. Patients often experience significant social, occupational, and personal consequences resulting from their picking behavior. At its most severe, Excoriation Disorder may be life-threatening (e.g., due to blood loss or septicemia) and require neurosurgical intervention (e.g., gamma knife capsulotomy has been used in a severe case).

While any part of the body can be picked, the most commonly endorsed area of picking is the face. Medical complications are common, and include infections, scarring, septicemia, and ulcerations. Skin Picking Disorder is common and more prevalent in females with prevalence rates ranging from 1.4–5.4% of the general population.

Excoriation Disorder appears to have a trimodal age of onset: in childhood (<10 years old), adolescence/early adulthood (15–21 years), and between the ages of 30–45. Excoriation Disorder is associated with a lower quality of life, reduced self-esteem, and avoidance of social situations due to shame and embarrassment resulting from the picking. The majority of affected individuals have never sought treatment or discussed their picking behaviors with healthcare professionals.

Diagnosis of Excoriation (Skin picking) Disorder

Excoriation Disorder has recently been included in the DSM-5 as a full disorder with criteria summarized as follows:

- Picking of the skin which results in wounds to the skin
- The person endorses trying to either cut back or stop picking
- The patient experiences distress as a result of skin picking or some aspect of social, work, or other area of functioning is impaired
- Drug use (such as amphetamine or cocaine) or a medical condition is not the cause of the skin picking
- Another mental health condition (such as picking to improve one's appearance or a perceived defect as seen in Body Dysmorphic Disorder, delusions or hallucinations, stereotypies, or international self-harm) is not the main prompt for skin picking

Although most people pick at their skin at some time, the above criteria differentiate typical and common picking from Excoriation Disorder. Most people who pick at their cuticles from time to time, for example, do not feel distressed by it and are not impaired due to the skin picking.

There are several questions that a clinician may use to assess the diagnostic criteria and to derive information regarding the picking behavior.

"Can you tell me why you pick?" This will help to rule out dermatological conditions and some psychiatric conditions.

"Can you control your picking?" or "Do you have urges to pick that are difficult for you to control?" Intense urges or tension or anxiety prior to actually engaging in the picking behavior are common in Excoriation Disorder and can potentially help in directing the patient for appropriate treatment.

"Are there activities or others things in your life that you avoid due to your picking?" Many patients will endorse not socializing with friends, refusing to wear short sleeves or shorts in the summer due to their scarring, or not dating because of their skin picking. It is reassuring for the patient to be able to tell someone about how picking affects their everyday life since many patients have been unable or unwilling to talk to someone about their picking before.

"At what time(s) in the day do you pick? For example, are you around other people or by yourself; do you pick most while driving or at home watching TV, etc.?"

"Do you have any triggers to your picking? For example, do you pick when you are tired, stressed, angry, sad, etc.?"

These questions can be beneficial when developing a behavioral therapy for the patient.

Scales

There are several valid and reliable measures/scales that can be used to monitor change in symptoms during treatment.

Scales have been developed in order to aid the clinician in assessing the severity of skin picking symptoms. These scales can be used to better understand the severity of the skin picking problem along with component parts of the picking such as the time spent having urges and thoughts to pick as well as time expended on the picking behavior itself.

Yale-Brown Obsessive Compulsive Scale, modified for Neurotic Excoriation (NE-YBOCS) is a modification of the Yale-Brown Obsessive Compulsive Scale, a 10-item clinician- administered scale for obsessive compulsive disorder. Picking symptoms are assessed during the last seven days on a severity scale from 0 to 4 for each item (total scores range from 0 to 40 with higher scores reflecting greater illness severity). The first five items of the NE-YBOCS comprise the picking urge/thought subscale (time occupied with urges/thoughts; interference and distress due to urges/thoughts; resistance against and control over urges/thoughts), and items 6–10 comprise the picking behavior subscale (time spent picking;

interference and distress due to picking; ability to resist and control picking behavior). The NE-YBOCS is particularly useful to examine the difference between urges/thoughts to pick and actual picking behavior.

Skin Picking Scale-Revised (SPS-R: Appendix C) is an 8-item, self-report measure for the assessment of skin picking. Individual scale items range from 0 to 4 with a total score range of 0 to 32. While a total score should be calculated, two subscale scores for "impairment" and "symptom severity" can also be calculated.

Skin Picking Self-Assessment Scale (SP-SAS) is a modification of a reliable and valid self-report scale used for other psychiatric disorders such as gambling disorder and kleptomania. The 12-item SP-SAS assesses picking urges, thoughts, and behaviors during the previous seven days. Each item is rated 0 to 4 with a possible total score of 48.

Milwaukee Inventory for the Dimensions of Adult Skin Picking (MIDAS) is a 12-item, self-report measure developed to distinguish between automatic (unconscious) and focused (conscious) picking of the skin. Each item is rated from 1 (not true of any of my skin picking) to 5 (true for all of my skin picking). This scale can help the clinician identify how aware each patient is of his/her skin picking as a means of potentially tailoring treatment to each individual. For example, individuals who are more automatic pickers may benefit from CBT awareness training.

Differential Diagnosis (or, When Is It Really Excoriation Disorder?)

Body Dysmorphic Disorder (BDD) is often the most difficult differential diagnosis to make. BDD is characterized by obsessions about and preoccupation with a perceived defect of physical appearance. A disproportionate obsession over perceived skin blemishes and subsequent picking at those areas can provide the clinician with a difficult task in establishing whether the picking is Excoriation Disorder or

BDD. In fact, some type of skin picking behavior occurs in between 26–45% of patients with BDD.

Ask the patient: "Are you very concerned about the appearance of some part(s) of your body that you consider particularly unattractive? And, if so, do these concerns preoccupy you?"

Ask the patient: "Do you pick your skin to improve the way you look?"

If "yes," the clinician should ask, "Regarding those places you pick to improve the way you look, do you feel there is something wrong with that/those body part(s)?"

If the patient answers "yes" to the above questions, the picking may be due to BDD and the rest of the BDD criteria should be examined.

Stimulant use: It is not uncommon for those that use or abuse stimulants (for example, cocaine, methamphetamine, and prescription stimulants) to excoriate the skin in response to skin sensations resulting from drug use. As such, stimulant use should be ruled out by the clinician. It is also possible that someone may have Excoriation Disorder which is worsened by stimulant use. In those cases, the picking may improve after stopping the stimulant but will most likely still remain in a less severe form.

Ask the patient: "Do you use any stimulants, either by prescription or recreationally?" If yes, "have you noticed any relationship between the use of the stimulant and your picking?"

Delusions of Parasitosis/Psychotic Disorder: It is important to distinguish between picking propagated by delusions or tactile hallucinations as seen in parasitosis where the individual is convinced (delusionally) that they are infested with a parasitic infection and may pick at their skin to uncover these parasites.

Ask the patient: "Can you tell me more about your motivation for picking? Do you pick to get to something underneath the skin?" If the patient reports that their skin has an infestation (or other wording) which he/she is picking to access, a psychotic disorder is the more likely diagnosis.

Obsessive Compulsive Disorder: Excessive washing compulsions in response to contamination obsessions in individuals with OCD may lead to skin lesions. In addition, individuals with contamination obsessions may also pick to remove particles of dirt or other contaminants from their skin.

Ask the patient: "Can you tell me more about your motivation for picking? Do you pick to clean your skin?" "Are you preoccupied with thoughts of being contaminated?"

Self-injury: Excoriation Disorder is not the same thing as self-injury. In fact, clinicians should not diagnose Excoriation Disorder if the skin picking is primarily attributable to the intention to harm oneself.

Ask the patient: "Do you pick at yourself to cause yourself pain? Possibly to deal with overwhelming emotions or situations, to feel in control or to stop feelings of numbness?"

If the person answers affirmatively to these questions, it may be important to examine other aspects of self-injury and/or to examine aspects of borderline personality disorder.

Other medical conditions: Excoriation Disorder should not be diagnosed if the skin picking is primarily attributable to a medical condition. For example, scabies is a dermatological condition invariably associated with severe itching and scratching. Excoriation Disorder, however, may be precipitated or exacerbated by an underlying dermatological condition. For example, acne may lead to some scratching and picking, which may also be associated with co-morbid Excoriation Disorder. The differentiation between these two clinical situations (acne with some scratching and picking versus acne with co-morbid Excoriation Disorder) requires an assessment of the extent to which the individual's skin picking has become independent of the underlying dermatological condition.

Ask the patient: "Although you started picking due to a skin condition, has the picking continued despite improvement in the skin condition? (Or) Does it seem that the picking has become its own independent problem?"

Co-morbidity and Sequencing Treatment

Co-morbid psychiatric conditions are extremely common in Excoriation Disorder and should always be screened for. Clinicians should start by ruling out psychiatric issues such as substance (especially amphetamine and cocaine) use or abuse which may worsen picking symptoms. The most common co-occurring conditions in Skin Picking Disorder include the following:

Trichotillomania. Approximately 38% of individuals with Excoriation Disorder have co-occurring Trichotillomania. Clinicians should understand and assess for the presence of Trichotillomania among those who present with Excoriation Disorder.

Obsessive Compulsive Disorder (OCD). Approximately 17% to 52% of individuals who present with Excoriation Disorder also have co-occurring OCD. The repetitive (compulsive) picking of the skin and obsessions over blemishes or making the skin feel "just right" illustrate the overlap between Excoriation Disorder and OCD and may complicate the clinical picture. While significant overlap exists between Excoriation Disorder and OCD, patients with Excoriation Disorder usually report that the urge to pick comes first, followed by finding the appropriate place on the body to pick. In addition, individuals with Excoriation Disorder often endorse a pleasurable affect from picking which is in stark contrast to engaging in OCD compulsions.

Major Depressive Disorder (MDD). MDD has been found in 26–31% of patients with Excoriation Disorder. It is not always clear if the depression is merely a consequence of the picking or an independent disorder. Determining a temporal relationship to the picking may be important to establish a treatment approach—for example, if the depression is clearly secondary to the picking, treatment could focus on picking.

Ideally, the clinician should treat both the skin picking and co-morbid condition simultaneously. Noteworthy exceptions include if the patient presents with symptoms of suicidality or psychotic symptoms which should be treated prior to treatment for any skin picking or other co-occurring condition.

Course and Prognosis

Excoriation Disorder usually has its onset in adolescence, commonly coinciding with or following the onset of puberty. The disorder frequently begins with a dermatological condition, such as acne. Sites of skin picking may vary over time. The usual course is chronic, with some waxing and waning if untreated. For some individuals, the disorder may come and go for weeks, months, or years at a time.

Individuals with excoriation are likely to present with other psychiatric ailments, including depression and/or anxiety as they may be unaware that Excoriation Disorder is a legitimate and treatable psychiatric condition. Most patients have told someone (loved one, friend, etc.) or been asked by someone (family member, friend) in the past about their picking but told to "just stop picking" or perceived the interaction as judgmental. Patients may perceive their picking as nothing more than a bad habit. As such, it is extremely important to directly ask the patient about any excoriations as they may be unlikely to endorse compulsive picking without prompting.

Treatment

Physical and Dermatological Examination

The clinical evaluation of someone with Excoriation Disorder entails a broad physical and psychiatric examination. The physical examination serves two purposes: first, to assess the extent of the picking and to develop appropriate interventions based on the damage to the skin (for example, does the person need antibiotics? Has a more systemic illness resulted from the picking such as bacteremia, cellulitis, or joint infection?); and second, to assess for possible dermatological or infectious etiologies of the skin picking.

In terms of the possible etiologies, there are many dermatological conditions that result in scratching or picking: scabies, atopic dermatitis, psoriasis, and blistering skin disorders to name only a few. Patients should be sent for a thorough dermatological consultation which may include microscopic examination of lesions for scabies, the Wood's lamp examination for fungal infections, patch testing for allergies, skin biopsies, and laboratory investigations of thyroid, parathyroid, liver, and kidney problems.

In children, the examination should also focus on the possibility that skin picking is associated with pervasive developmental disorders or Prader-Willi Syndrome. Prader-Willi syndrome is a rare genetic disorder that is often associated with hyperphagia, hypogonadism, and frequent skin picking. Picking in individuals with Prader-Willi or with developmental disabilities may require specialized treatment interventions, such as combinations of differential reinforcement, providing preferred items and activities (e.g., toys), wearing protective clothing (e.g., helmets or gloves), and response interruption and redirection.

Psychotherapy

Cognitive Behavioral Therapy (CBT) techniques are the most widely recognized treatment for Excoriation Disorder although the specific duration of treatment is unknown at this time and likely varies from patient to patient. Early CBT treatment studies provide preliminary evidence for skin picking reduction with habit reversal or acceptance-enhanced behavior therapy.

Habit Reversal Therapy (HRT) is a first-line treatment and focuses on awareness training (encouraging awareness of situations that can precede picking episodes); relaxation training (since anxiety and stress are commonly reported triggers for skin picking episodes); competing response training (encouraging unwanted picking behaviors to be replaced with a less conspicuous action—e.g., clenching fists or squeezing a stress ball antagonistic to the picking action); social support (someone who can point out the person's behavior to help him or her become more aware and to remind the patient to practice the competing response); motivation procedures (designed to improve how acceptable HRT is to patients and their families); and generalization training (rehearsing trigger situations and the sequence of starting the picking episode, quelling it, and undertaking a competing response). There is evidence that a short course of HRT (3–6 sessions) may be beneficial.

Stress reduction training, in conjunction with habit reversal techniques, are also beneficial in helping patients to reduce picking and deal with emotion regulation difficulties. Depending on the triggers of the patient, learning how to reduce stress may alleviate some of the intensity of picking urges and behavior. For example, if the patient reports that high levels of work stress generally trigger a picking episode in the car on the way home from the office, the clinician can suggest ideas to manage the stress without picking (such as going for a vigorous walk immediately after work prior to getting in the car).

Acceptance and Commitment Therapy (ACT) is a therapy technique in which patients are asked to experience urges to pick and accept the urge without acting on it. The negative emotions involved with picking are also engaged but not acted upon. The idea is that understanding, feeling, and experiencing the fact that the individuals do not have to respond to an urge or emotion can help the patient to feel more in control of their picking. ACT has generally involved 8 sessions to treat Excoriation Disorder although a shorter or longer duration of therapy sessions may be indicated based upon patient symptoms and preference.

Online Therapy. Online therapeutic tools have also been developed by expert clinicians with a substantial amount of experience treating skin picking, including at www.stoppicking.com. The behavioral therapy offered online seeks to help the patient to identify situations or triggers prompting skin picking and subsequently strategize ways in which the patient can address and change those behaviors. Online therapy has been reported as particularly useful for individuals living in rural communities, those with a hectic schedule, or for those who prefer to engage in therapy without leaving their home (due to, for example, embarrassment or shame from lesions or scars resulting from where skin picking has occurred).

Pharmacotherapy

There are no labeled medications for the treatment of Excoriation Disorder and research into pharmacotherapeutic efficacy for Excoriation Disorder is relatively limited at this time.

Data regarding the efficacy of serotonin reuptake inhibitors has been mixed. Based on the research, fluoxetine (target dose of 60mg/day), citalopram (target dose of 20mg/day), and escitalopram (target dose of 25mg/day) may all be somewhat beneficial for Excoriation Disorder.

The opioid antagonist, naltrexone (50mg/day) has demonstrated some benefit for Excoriation Disorder, as has the glutamatergic agent *n*-acetylcysteine (NAC) (1,800mg/day); however, these medications have been used in small samples of patients. Adult patients with Skin Picking Disorder should start treatment with *n*-acetylcysteine at 600mg twice/day for one week, then 1,200mg twice/day for up to four weeks, and then 1,800mg upon awakening and 1,200mg about 10 hours later per day.

Initiation/Ongoing Treatment

Baseline investigations are not needed before starting SSRIs or NAC. If someone responds to an SSRI or NAC, a course of treatment should be for at least one year. Similarly, if depression or anxiety is co-occurring, SSRI medication management for at least one year may be necessary. In cases where the patient presents with suicidal ideation or plan, appropriate clinical interventions should be made prior to treating the skin picking symptoms.

Baseline investigations prior to initiation of naltrexone should include liver function tests. These should be repeated at 3 and 6 months, then at 1 year, then annually thereafter (unless there are specific concerns).

Before starting psychotherapy, the clinician should make sure the patient (and family, in the case of children) knows the intended number of therapy sessions and the need to perform homework assignments.

Risks/Side Effects

The clinically most common side effects from *n*-acetylcysteine include nausea, indigestion, headache, and abdominal pain although it is generally well tolerated. Contraindications include current asthma and current pregnancy/lactation as the effects of NAC on fetal development has not been assessed.

The clinically most common side effects from SSRI medications include nausea, dry mouth, headache, diarrhea, nervousness, agitation or restlessness, reduced sexual desire or difficulty reaching orgasm, inability to maintain an erection (erectile dysfunction), rash, increased sweating, weight gain, drowsiness, or insomnia.

The most common adverse events resulting from naltrexone include nausea, sedation, vivid dreaming, and dizziness. Rarer but a more serious side effect of naltrexone may include elevated liver function tests (LFTs). If this occurs, the medication should be stopped and LFTs monitor until they return to baseline. Use of other the counter analgesics may increase the likelihood for elevated LFTs. Naltrexone should not be started in anyone who is taking opioid agonists.

Adolescent and young adult patients with excoriation and co-occurring Major Depressive Disorder or symptoms of depression who are taking antidepressant medications should be alerted to the risk of clinical worsening of depressive symptoms and suicidal ideation which have been linked to the use of these medications. Parents and guardians of children who are prescribed antidepressants, regardless of depression history, should be alerted to this risk.

Treatment Choice and Sequencing of Treatment

If untreated, Excoriation Disorder is a chronic illness that often results in substantial psychosocial dysfunction and may lead to medical complications. Control of the skin picking is therefore critical for maintaining long-term health and quality of life. Based on our clinical experience and research findings, we suggest the following management strategies:

- Begin with a thorough psychiatric assessment to establish an accurate diagnosis of Excoriation Disorder and to assess for co-occurring psychiatric disorders;
- Thorough evaluation from a dermatologist with knowledge about Excoriation Disorder to assess for underlying dermatological conditions that may cause or worsen skin picking;
- Maintain collaboration between internal medicine and psychiatric management teams for monitoring and rapid intervention if serious medical sequelae result from the picking;
- Provide education about the disorder to the patient, including possible etiologies, and treatment risks and benefits; and
- Provide CBT (including habit reversal or acceptance-enhanced behavior therapy) as first-line treatment for Excoriation Disorder.

Given the relative paucity of information regarding a treatment of choice for Excoriation Disorder, medications (serotonin reuptake inhibitors, *n*-acetylcysteine, or naltrexone) or techniques used in CBT may be used as monotherapies or in conjunction with one another. Choice of medication should be informed by the existence of co-occurring disorders and patient history. SSRIs may be the first choice if the patient has co-occurring depression or anxiety whereas NAC may be the first choice for someone with no co-occurring disorders. Naltrexone may be the choice for someone with a personal or family history of addictions.

Consultation with Other Disciplines

Dermatologic consultation should occur where significant inflammation of the skin occurs at the site of picking, or where there is diagnostic uncertainty as to the cause of the skin picking. Consultation with dermatological colleagues can also be helpful where an individual endorses sensations on the skin that prompt picking episodes.

Clinical Pearls for Excoriation (Skin Picking) Disorder

- Habit reversal therapy is the psychotherapy of choice.
- Medication options are unclear at this time although many people benefit from pharmacotherapy.
- Excoriation Disorder is often co-morbid with Trichotillomania, Body Dysmorphic Disorder, OCD, and major depression.
- Skin picking may have origins in other psychiatric conditions, including illicit substance use (methamphetamine), Body Dysmorphic Disorder, delusions of parasitosis, all of which must be ruled out.
- Infections resulting from skin picking are common and patients may require antibiotic or, in severe cases, surgical intervention.

Key References

- Odlaug BL, Grant JE. Pathologic skin picking. Am J Drug Alcohol Abuse. 2010 Sep;36(5):296–303.
- Tucker BT, Woods DW, Flessner CA, Franklin SA, Franklin ME. The Skin Picking Impact Project: phenomenology, interference, and treatment utilization of pathological skin picking in a population-based sample. J Anxiety Disord. 2011 Jan;25(1):88–95.
- Grant JE, Odlaug BL, Chamberlain SR, Keuthen NJ, Lochner C, Stein J. Skin picking disorder. Am J Psychiatry. 2012 Nov 1;169(11):1143–9.

9

Tic Disorders

Clinical Description

Tics are repetitive, brief, jerky motor movements and/or vocalizations. Any part of the body can be affected but common visible sites include the face (e.g. blinking, grimacing, chin-protruding, clearing one's throat, or making other vocalizations) and upper body (e.g., moving one's neck to the side, shoulder, and limb movements). The assessment of tics can be difficult as they naturally wax and wane over time, and are also commonplace in a subclinical form, especially in young people. In fact, one of the authors of this book was trained to look for subtle perinasal tics by an experienced OCD psychiatrist when he was a medical student, and now sees tics wherever he goes. While subclinical tics are common (up to 15% of children), however, formal Tic Disorders are more rare, ranging from 0.5% (Tourette's Syndrome) through to up to 6% (Transient Tic Disorder) in children and adolescents. Adult Tic Disorders are considerably rarer.

Motor tics typically precede vocal tics by one or two years, and tics in general peak during late childhood and adolescence (aged 10–20 years), often with a marked reduction in severity into early adulthood. Where tics start in adulthood (a form of Tic Disorder not otherwise specified), symptoms are more functionally impairing and difficult to treat. Tics can increase during times of extreme emotion, and reduce with voluntary effort (in some individuals) and when concentrating on intricate tasks. They can be preceded by sensory experiences or urges and followed by relief.

Diagnosis

The DSM-5 Diagnostic Criteria for Tic Disorders distinguishes three types of condition: Tourette's Disorder, Persistent Tic Disorder, and Provisional Tic Disorder. There are also the options of diagnosing "Other Specified Tic Disorder" or "Unspecified Tic Disorder" where full criteria are not met.

The main diagnostic aspects can be distilled down as follows:

- For any tic-related diagnosis, there must be significant functional impairment and symptoms must not be due to a medical condition or physiological effects of substance.
- Tic free periods are permissible and it is recognized that tics do wax and wane—this does not prevent a diagnosis being made.
- The occurrence of one or more tics, persisting for <1 year, with initial onset in childhood, gives a diagnosis of Provisional Tic Disorder.
- The occurrence of one or more tics, persisting for >1 year, with initial onset in childhood, gives a diagnosis of either:
  - Tourette's Disorder where there have been several motor tics and at least one vocal tic at some point; or
  - Persistent Tic Disorder otherwise (can specify "with motor tics only" or "with vocal tics only")
- If there are symptoms of a Tic Disorder causing significant functional impairment but full diagnostic criteria are not met for the above, then the diagnosis of Other Specified Tic Disorder or Unspecified Tic Disorder can be considered. The former is where the clinician wishes to specify the reason full criteria are not met (e.g., adult onset tics), while the latter is where no explicit explanation is yet given (e.g., where information collection is ongoing).

TABLE 9.1 Terminology Used for DSM-5 and ICD-10 for Tic Disorders

DSM-5	ICD-10
Provisional Tic Disorder	Transient Tic Disorder
Persistent Tic Disorder	Chronic Motor or Vocal Tic Disorder
Tourette's Disorder	Combined Tic Disorder
Other Specified Tic Disorder/ Unspecified Tic Disorder	Tic Disorder, Unspecified

The ICD-10 (see Table 9.1 for equivalent disorders between the two diagnostic systems) is also slightly more prescriptive in terms of criteria that must be met:

- Transient Tic Disorder: Tic(s) occur many times a day, most days, for at least four weeks.
- Chronic Motor or Vocal Tic Disorder: Tic(s) occur many times a day, most days, over a period of at least 12 months.
- Combined Tic Disorder: Tics occur many times a day, nearly every day for more than one year, with no period of remission during that year lasting longer than two months.
- Tic Disorder, unspecified, is utilized for individuals with tics that do not clearly fall into the above three categories and/or where full criteria are not met.

Co-morbidity

As a starting point, the clinician should screen suitably for the presence of pervasive developmental disorders such as autism, and learning disability (low intelligence quotient, IQ) which can present with stereotyped and ritualistic behavior, in addition to tics. These are unlikely in those presenting with tics as the primary symptom but should not be missed.

Attention Deficit Hyperactivity Disorder. Problems with inattention, hyperactivity, and/or impulsivity are frequent in people with Tic Disorders. It can be difficult clinically to discern the diagnostic boundaries, particularly given that Attention Deficit Hyperactivity Disorder (ADHD) is quite difficult to objectively diagnose. Up to 50% of people with Tic Disorders meet diagnostic criteria for co-morbid ADHD. The diagnosis of ADHD is outside the scope of this guide.

Obsessive Compulsive Disorder. Subclinical obsessive compulsive symptoms are common in people with Tic Disorders, and up to 50% of patients with Tic Disorders have co-morbid formal OCD. Obsessive compulsive symptoms often begin to occur later than tics (average 1–2 years later). While any OCD symptoms can occur, the most frequent obsessions in people with tic spectrum disorders include those of an aggressive, sexual, and religious nature, while the most common compulsions include ordering-up, counting, and making sure things are "just right."

Other co-morbid psychiatric disorders to be on guard for in people with Tic Disorders include depression and anxiety disorders (each found in approximately 10–15% of patients).

Course and Prognosis

There is considerable variability in the onset and time course of Tic Disorders. Motor tics commonly start around 3–8 years of age, and vocal tics start several years later (if they co-occur). Tics tend to worsen initially, peaking in severity at a mean age of 10 years old, and subsequently declining in severity over time with 50–90% of individuals exhibiting no or minimal tics by adulthood. In a given individual, tics wax and wane considerably over time, which can make it difficult to address whether a particular treatment is working effectively for that person or not.

Children with Tic Disorders show psychosocial impairment, although the relationship with tic severity is disputed, and in many cases impairment appears to be more driven by co-morbid ADHD rather than tics themselves. Long-term functional outcomes in children with Tic Disorders followed into adulthood are not well studied; there is some evidence that a degree of functional impairment can persist even with symptoms becoming less severe, at least into early adulthood. Adults with chronic Tic Disorders also show lower quality of life and mild-moderate functional impairment (e.g., avoidance of social events and public places, interference in work activities, interference in relationships). It is also known that for individuals first showing tics as adults, symptoms are harder to treat and more likely to persist with advancing age.

Differential Diagnosis (or, When Is a Tic Not a Tic?)

Tics are brief non-rhythmic "jerky" movements and vocalizations. Bear in mind the following types of abnormal movements, which can masquerade as tics:

- *Blepharospasm.* Focal contraction of muscles around the eyes—commonplace involuntary movement, often incorrectly described as a tic.
- *Akathesia.* A sense of inner restlessness, relieved by moving about, e.g., marching, rocking, or squirming. Akathesia can occur due to antipsychotic medication, especially at high doses or when newly introduced.
- *Tremor.* An involuntary, rhythmic type of movement that can be primary (essential tremor) or secondary (e.g., due to medications/drugs, Parkinson's Disease, or metabolic disturbance).
- *Athetosis.* Slow, writhing, continuous movements (e.g., in cerebral palsy).

- *Dystonia.* Continuous unwanted contractions of muscles, which are often painful (e.g., due to nerve compression, or as a reaction to antipsychotics).
- *Chorea.* Irregular random "dance like" sets of movements, abrupt and un-sustained, but seeming to flow from one body part to another. Unpredictable in timing, direction, and body part affected (e.g., Sydenham's Chorea; e.g., Huntington's Disease).
- *Tardive dyskinesia.* Repetitive movements occurring due to chronic antipsychotic use (especially first generation)—includes grimacing, smacking one's lips, rapid eye blinks, and tongue protrusion

The differentiation of tics from these other types of movement is greatly aided by observation of abnormal movements themselves (where possible) and by taking a detailed psychiatric history, which should include questions about exacerbating and relieving factors, prescribed medications, past medical history (such as of childhood streptococcal infection), and any salient family history (neurologic and psychiatric conditions in first-degree relatives).

Monitoring Treatment

It can be helpful to monitor over a period of months to assess tic fluctuation and gauge impact of tics on school, social, and family functioning:

The Yale Global Tic Severity Scale (YGTSS: Appendix C) is a recommended instrument for documenting the nature and severity of tics, and treatment response. It is a clinician-administered instrument and is suitable for the assessment of child and adult patients. The **YGTSS** considers, for motor and vocal tics: number, frequency, intensity, complexity, and interference. This yields a total tic (motor + vocal) severity score of 0–50, based on symptoms over the past week. The total tic severity scores can be broadly categorized as: no tics (0), minimal tics (0–9), mild tics (11–19), and moderate-severe tics (>19). We recommend that treatment response be defined as a

35% or greater reduction in total tic severity score. The **YGTSS** TS also includes an "impairment" scale of 0–50, ranging from minimal impairment to severe impairment.

Treatment

In a minority of cases, individuals with tics may present due to friends or relatives being concerned, rather than any distress from the affected individual; in such cases, treatment may not be needed. In the case of new, subtle, or non-distressing tics, it may be appropriate to take a "watchful waiting" approach, with outpatient follow-up, and consideration of treatment at a later date.

Before rushing in with specific treatment for the Tic Disorder itself, consider whether co-morbid disorders are present, and treat these as a priority. This is particularly important for co-morbid OCD and ADHD, where treatment of these symptoms may have beneficial effects on tics, too.

Pharmacotherapy

Antipsychotic medications are regarded as the most effective established pharmacological treatment for tics, although their side effect profiles are problematic and hinder their clinical use. The antipsychotic medications studied most for the treatment of Tic Disorders are: risperidone, pimozide, and haloperidol. Aripiprazole has also been explored but further controlled trials are needed.

The alpha-2 receptor agonist medications clonidine and guanfacine also show efficacy in the treatment of tics, and were traditionally recommended over-and-above antipsychotics, due to their superior side effect profiles. However, recent meta-analysis suggests that alpha-2 receptor agonists are only of significant clinical benefit when used in patients with Tic Disorder plus ADHD, rather than Tic Disorder alone.

Adult dosing guidelines are as follows (for doses in children/adolescents see the relevant section elsewhere in this book):

- Risperidone: Start with 0.5 or 1mg per day, and increase at intervals of 2–7 days in steps of 0.5–1mg per day, depending on progress. The mean effective dose is 3mg. Suggested maximum 6mg per day. Can be given once daily or in two divided doses.
- Pimozide: Start with 1mg per day, and increase at intervals of 1mg per day every 2–7 days, depending on progress. The mean effective dose is 3mg per day. Suggested maximum 6mg per day.
- Haloperidol: Start with 0.5mg per day, and increase at intervals of 2–7 days in steps of 0.5mg per day, depending on symptom response and tolerability. Suggested maximum dose is 3mg per day.
- Clonidine: Start with 50 micrograms twice each day, increasing after two weeks to 75 micrograms twice each day (if needed) and if physical observations are acceptable (blood pressure and pulse).
- Guanfacine: Start with 1mg per day, and increase at intervals of one week by 0.5–1mg per day, depending on response, and if physical observations are acceptable (blood pressure and pulse). Recommended maximum 4mg/day.

Indications/Efficacy

In general, we recommend psychotherapy if available (see below) rather than pharmacotherapy as the first-line treatment for Tic Disorders. Where there is insufficient clinical response to an appropriate course of psychotherapy, or where symptoms are severely disabling, antipsychotic medication can be considered, after careful evaluation and discussion with the patient of the positive and negatives associated with particular antipsychotic medication treatment. The threshold for prescribing antipsychotics is lower in adults due to more safety data being available, and knowledge that adult Tic Disorders are more functionally impairing and persistent than the childhood onset form.

In the special case of moderate to severe Tic Disorder plus ADHD, we recommend an alpha-2 receptor agonist (clonidine or guanfacine) as a first-line option for children and adults, in addition to psychotherapy.

Initiation/Ongoing Treatment

Baseline investigations prior to initiation of antipsychotic medication should include an EKG (ECG), fasting lipid levels and glucose, liver function tests, urea and electrolytes, full blood count, and prolactin; pulse and blood pressure should be recorded along with body mass index and waist circumference. These should be repeated at 6 months, then at 1 year, then annually thereafter (unless there are specific concerns).

Before starting an alpha-2 receptor agonist, an EKG (ECG) should be undertaken; blood pressure and pulse should also be recorded. Following any dose increases, it is prudent to repeat these investigations.

Before starting psychotherapy, the clinician should make sure the patient (and family, in the case of children) knows the intended number of therapy sessions, and the need to perform homework assignments.

Risks/Side Effects

The clinically most common side effects from antipsychotic medications include: sedation, weight gain, elevated lipids / glucose, and constipation.

Rarer but serious side effects of antipsychotics include: extrapyramidal side effects (including acute dystonic reactions), neuroleptic malignant syndrome (NMS), drug-induced Parkinsonism, dry mouth, blurred vision, elevated prolactin (which can lead to sexual dysfunction in men and women), urinary retention, and clinically significant EKG (ECG) changes, e.g., QT prolongation.

The clinically most common side effects from alpha-1 receptor agonists include: initial sedation, postural hypotension, constipation, and mid-sleep wakening (although overall, these medications can be helpful for sleep disturbances). Guanfacine appears to have less risk of sedation than clonidine.

Rarer but serious side effects of alpha-1 receptor agonists include: low mood. Additionally, patients should be warned that alpha-1 agonists should not be stopped abruptly due to risk of rebound syndrome (hypertension, anxiety, tremor, palpitations, and muscular pain).

Psychotherapy

Habit Reversal Therapy (HRT) is relatively well established in the treatment of Tic Disorders, with large effect size versus control conditions. HRT is first-line treatment focusing on: awareness training (encouraging awareness of situations that can precede tics and awareness of the nature of the tics); relaxation training (since anxiety and stress can trigger tics); competing response training (encouraging unwanted tics to be replaced with a less conspicuous action—e.g., tensing muscles antagonistic to the tic action); motivation procedures (designed to improve how acceptable HRT is to patients and their families); and generalization training (rehearsing trigger situations and the sequence of starting the tic, stopping it, and undertaking a competing response). There is evidence that a short course of HRT is as effective as more protracted number of sessions; and that benefits extend beyond the end of the treatment.

Exposure and Response Prevention (ERP) also shows efficacy in the treatment of Tic Disorders, and involves exposure to sensations and urges preceding tics, and response prevention of the tics. In a head-to-head comparison, ERP and HRT were similarly effective for tic symptoms, but it should be noted that ERP is typically more involving in terms of therapist/patient time.

Treatment Choice and Sequencing of Treatment

Psychological therapy (HRT or ERP) should be implemented as a first-line treatment for Tic Disorders where treatment is indicated.

For those with severely functionally impairing tics, and for those who cannot engage with psychological therapy, antipsychotic medication can be considered. Likewise, tics that persist and impair life despite a course of talk therapy can be treated with antipsychotic medication. For patients with Tic Disorder plus ADHD, an alpha-2 receptor agonist (clonidine or guanfacine) should be started as the first-line treatment in conjunction with psychotherapy: this is important since these two conditions likely have synergistic negative effects on long-term functional outcomes if not robustly treated.

Clinical Pearls for Tic Disorders

- Carefully explore the tic description to help rule out other tic-like movements (e.g. chorea, tardive dyskinesia).
- Highly co-morbid with ADHD, OCD, depression, and anxiety disorders.
- For tics, watchful waiting is often appropriate, especially when the patient is not unduly concerned about tics themselves or is not grossly functionally impaired. Where treatment is indicated, psychological therapy (habit reversal therapy and/or exposure and response prevention) is first-line.
- In moderate-severe Tic Disorders, or where psychological treatment fails, medication should be considered: start with an antipsychotic except in the case of co-morbid ADHD, where an alpha-2 receptor agonist should be used (clonidine or guanfacine).

Key References

- Knight T, Steeves T, Day L, Lowerison M, Jette N, Pringsheim T. Prevalence of tic disorders: a systematic review and meta-analysis. Pediatr Neurol. 2012 Aug;47(2):77–90.

- Weisman H, Qureshi IA, Leckman JF, Scahill L, Bloch MH. Systematic review: pharmacological treatment of tic disorders—efficacy of antipsychotic and alpha-2 adrenergic agonist agents. Neurosci Biobehav Rev. 2013 Jul;37(6):1162–71.
- Wile DJ, Pringsheim TM. Behavior Therapy for Tourette Syndrome: A Systematic Review and Meta-analysis. Curr Treat Options Neurol. 2013 Aug;15(4):385–95.

PART THREE

SPECIAL CLINICAL CONSIDERATIONS

10

Special Issues in Treatment

Treatment Resistant Cases

A number of patients with OCD and related disorders do not show adequate response to usual first-line psychological and pharmacological interventions.

As a broad rule we would recommend that "treatment resistance" be defined as a failure to respond to at least two adequate courses of evidence-based pharmacotherapies and at least one adequate course of evidence-based psychotherapy. Failure to respond can be operationalized as less than 25–35% reduction in total symptom severity scores as compared to the pre-treatment baseline. By way of example, for Obsessive Compulsive Disorder (OCD), treatment resistance would be less than 25–35% reduction in total Yale-Brown Obsessive Compulsive Scale (YBOCS) scores (versus pre-treatment baseline) following a course of two Serotonin Reuptake Inhibitors (SRIs) (each of at least 6 week duration at a therapeutic doses), and a minimum 12 session (12 hour) course of manualized validated Cognitive Behavioral Therapy (CBT) with Exposure and Response Prevention (ERP).

In possible treatment-resistant cases, the following steps can be very useful:

1. Re-evaluate the symptom history and presentation to confirm not only that any diagnoses are correct, but also that other diagnoses (including personality disorders) have not been overlooked. In considering this, do not forget to ask about Substance Use Disorders (alcohol, smoking, illicit substances), and medical conditions. See the individual disorder chapters

for lists of common differential diagnoses and co-morbidities for each OC Family Disorder.

2. Take a detailed history of treatments received to date, wherever possible in conjunction with case note review. If medications were received, were they titrated to therapeutic doses? Did patients receive therapeutic doses for a reasonable treatment duration (such as minimum six weeks for SRI treatment of OCD)? Check with patients about any side effects they noticed and sensitively ask whether they were compliant with a given medication consistently over the course of the intervention. For psychotherapy, check about attendance, content, length of each session, number of sessions received, and who conducted the therapy. Were there any difficulties that stopped the patient being able to engage with a given therapy? Again, the clinician should look to evaluate whether any psychological treatments received were adequate in order to conclude that a given modality was ineffective.
3. Assess for any predisposing, precipitating, and perpetuating factors. Exploring perpetuating factors in particular could help to identify reasons for treatment non-response and identify modifiable contributing factors. For example, there may be psychosocial stressors (difficult family dynamics or a stressful job situation). It can be helpful to ask about any first-degree relatives with psychiatric conditions and what treatments worked for them. For example, there may have been a parent with OCD who responded well to a given medication: if so, has this medication been tried in the patient?
4. In light of the above, consider:
    a. Pharmacological and psychological augmentation strategies (see disorder specific chapters for lists of treatment options in refractory cases where known)
    b. Use of inpatient management (see section later in this chapter on Hospitalization, Day Treatments, and Residential Treatments)

c. Referring the patient to more specialized services for consideration of other treatment strategies including the use of psychosurgery or deep brain stimulation where indicated and an evidence base exists (see section later in this chapter on Neurosurgery for OCD)
d. Suggesting to patients that they try alternative treatments in addition to evidence based treatments (see Alternative Treatments section later in this chapter)

Key References

- Abudy A, Juven-Wetzler A, Zohar J. Pharmacological management of treatment-resistant obsessive compulsive disorder. CNS Drugs. 2011 Jul;25(7):585–96.
- Boschen MJ, Drummond LM, Pillay A, Morton K. Predicting outcome of treatment for severe, treatment resistant OCD in inpatient and community settings. J Behav Ther Exp Psychiatry. 2010 Jun;41(2):90–5.
- Dold M, Aigner M, Lanzenberger R, Kasper S. Antipsychotic augmentation of serotonin reuptake inhibitors in treatment-resistant obsessive compulsive disorder: a meta-analysis of double-blind, randomized, placebo-controlled trials. Int J Neuropsychopharmacol. 2013 Apr;16(3):557–74.

Special Issues in Detection and Treatment of Childhood Disorders

Children and Adolescents

Several of the Obsessive Compulsive Related disorders are relatively common in childhood. For many adult patients seen in clinic, the onset of original psychopathology was in childhood but the disorder was missed for years by clinicians. Prompt treatment intervention in childhood may well stem the progression and impact of the illness. Most psychiatric research has been conducted in adults; and psychopathology in children can be quite difficult to disentangle.

OCD has a bimodal distribution in terms of age of onset, with one of the peaks being in childhood (12–14 years) and the other in early adulthood (20 years). OCD prevalence in children (1–4%) is similar to that in adults, that is, fairly commonplace.

Hoarding Disorder occurs in 1–2% of children, and rates of co-morbidity in such individuals are not well characterized: some studies even suggest that children with Hoarding Disorder do not show elevated rates of co-morbidity versus unaffected children. In children with OCD or ADHD, hoarding symptoms are common, occurring in up to one-third of patients. In childhood OCD, co-morbid hoarding is associated with worse insight, higher levels of aggression and anxiety/somatic complaints, higher rates of Panic Disorder, more magical thinking obsessions, and more ordering/arranging compulsions. In childhood ADHD, co-morbid hoarding is associated with more severe ADHD symptoms. Children with learning disability show elevated rates of hoarding (16% of cases), and where both diagnoses exist, ADHD (50%) and OCD (30%) are very frequent.

Childhood prevalence of *Body Dysmorphic Disorder (BDD)* is not known, but may be similar to that found in adults (0.5–1%), with onset typically occurring in the teenage years, not helped by media focus on body image.

Illness Anxiety Disorder (Hypochondriasis) is very rare in children, but medically unexplained physical symptoms are common and can signify other underlying psychiatric illnesses (e.g., anxiety disorders) or family stressors. Where Hypochondriasis is suspected in a child, consider the family dynamics: there may be excess concern from parents contributing to the child's complaints, or the child may have experienced a close family member developing a serious illness such as cancer.

Trichotillomania, the archetypal grooming disorder, commonly begins in adolescence (peak onset at 12–13 years of age), and 1–3% of adolescents have the disorder. When Trichotillomania occurs in very young children (4 years and below), it can resolve spontaneously with time and pharmacological treatment may not be indicated (though psychotherapy can be considered). The most common co-morbidities in childhood Trichotillomania include: anxiety disorders (30–60%), and ADHD (30%).

The prevalence of *Excoriation (Skin Picking) Disorder* in children is not known, although 10–40% of children pick their skin to some degree, suggesting that the pathological form is unlikely to be rare. Adults with childhood onset skin picking behaviors show less awareness of symptoms. Little is known of rates of co-morbidities between Excoriation Disorder and other conditions in childhood.

The majority of *Tic Disorders* begin before adulthood, as recognized by the inclusion of "onset before 18 years" in the diagnostic criteria (for all Tic Disorders except Other Specified Tic Disorder/ Unspecified Tic Disorder in DSM-5). It has been estimated that up to 8% of children have Tic Disorders, with peak onset at 5–7 years of age. Chronic Tic Disorders occur in 0.3–1.3% of youths. Most common co-morbidities include ADHD (40–70%), OCD (40–55%), learning disability (20–30%), and anxiety/mood disorders (18–30%).

Assessment

Each child or adolescent case requires a detailed assessment—more time is needed than for adult assessments. When possible, always ask the parents about pregnancy, birth, subsequent developmental milestones, and education (where relevant). Carefully explore the nature of any symptoms (including due consideration of co-morbidities) and their impact in different settings, but also take note of psychosocial and family context. In older children and adolescents, do not forget to sensitively ask about alcohol and illicit drug use. Where possible, interview the older child separately from family members, and then with family members. This gives the opportunity to sensitively ask the child about the possibility of any abuse (e.g., "Are you scared of anyone trying to hurt you? Does anyone hurt you at home or school?")

There may also be family pressures to obtain a specific diagnosis for the child in question and sensitivities from parents about whether the child's problems are "their fault." It is important to allay these fears and to explain at the outset that before any diagnosis is considered, you will need to take a detailed history not only from the child but also from those who know them. Also explain that not all inappropriate or unwanted behaviors in children mean that there is an underlying psychiatric condition.

Diagnosis

Check whether medical records and developmental history are suggestive of underlying genetic disorders or medical conditions. Key genetic disorders to consider include:

- *Fragile X Syndrome*. This genetic disorder is due to an excess of CGG repeats on the X chromosome, in a region coding for the "Fragile X mental retardation 1" or "FMR1" gene. This leads to abnormality in the expression of a protein involved in brain development. Characteristic features include intellectual disability, elongated face, large/protruding ears, and/or large testes. Fragile X syndrome is associated with *repetitive movements* (e.g., hand-flapping, head-banging, skin-picking), autism, and social anxiety.
- *Down Syndrome*. This is a genetic condition (extra copy of all or part of chromosome 21) and the most common genetic cause of learning disability. Common physical characteristics include reduced muscle tone, single creases in palms, upslanting palpebral fissures, and oversized tongue. ADHD symptoms are very common in Down syndrome.
- *Prader-Willi Syndrome*. This is a relatively rare genetic condition causing a wide range of features, including learning disability, extreme food intake, short stature, and reduced muscle tone. Compulsive behaviors, especially skin-picking, are commonplace, as is anxiety. People with Prader-Willi Syndrome may hoard items, especially food.

The above list is not exhaustive. Where the clinical presentation/physical features of any child raise suspicion of a genetic disorder, you should strongly consider referring the individual to a specialist—especially to a pediatrician and geneticist.

Consider the following psychiatric developmental disorders in relation to co-morbidities and differential diagnosis, in addition to those you would usually consider for the suspected OC disorder:

- *Intellectual Difficulties*. Where your history taking and interview suggest pronounced and widespread problems in general mental abilities, consider the possibility of an underlying Intellectual Difficulty. This is confirmed by formal cognitive testing (impairment more than two standard deviations below the matched population mean, i.e., IQ <75) and where the impairment affects adaptive everyday functioning.
- *Attention Deficit Hyperactivity Disorder* (ADHD; DSM-5), also known as *Hyperkinetic Disorder* (ICD-10). This is one of the most common psychiatric disorders of childhood. The hallmark is the occurrence of persistent problems of inattention and/or hyperactivity-impulsivity, some of which were present before the age of twelve years. The symptoms impact at least two distinct functional domains (e.g., schooling and socializing). Collateral information (e.g., from school teachers and parents) is particularly important in order to confirm this diagnosis.
- *Autism Spectrum Disorder* (ASD). Individuals with ASD show impaired social communication *and* social interactions *and* have a restricted range of interests/behaviors. Symptoms must begin in early childhood and impact everyday functioning.
- *Stereotypic Movement Disorder*. Individuals undertake repetitive purposeless behaviors such as body rocking, head banging, biting one's self, and hand shaking. This commonly exists in learning disabled individuals. The movements interfere with functioning and usually start in early development. Be careful to only utilize this diagnosis where symptoms are not better accounted for by another diagnosis. For example, circumscribed repetitive hair pulling in the absence

of other repetitive movements should be diagnosed as Trichotillomania rather than Stereotypic Movement Disorder.

- *Pediatric Autoimmune Neuropsychiatric Disorders Associated with Streptococcal Infection* (PANDAS). This condition is rare. The hallmark is prepubertal sudden and rapid onset of OC symptoms (e.g., OCD, tics), in association with beta-hemolytic streptococcal infection. Symptoms alter in nature and severity remarkably quickly, and there are often abnormalities on neurologic examination. There may be an elevated antistreptolysin O titer, which can suggest current or past streptococcal infection. Sequelae of rheumatic fever should be considered (polyarthritis, endocarditis, subcutaneous nodules, erythema marginatum, Sydenham's chorea). See the disorder-relevant section on PANDAS for more details.

Treatment

The treatment of pediatric patients should be guided by input from specialists in child and adolescent psychiatry. Treatment sequencing depends on a careful assessment of benefits and risks, and patient/family choice, bearing in mind the available evidence. Be careful to clearly document any treatment decisions and that you have fully discussed benefits and risks with the parent(s) or guardian(s), and patient as appropriate in light of their age.

As a general principle, when a patient has a co-morbid moderate-severe depressive or anxiety disorder, focus on treating that first (rather than the OC spectrum disorder). OC symptoms often improve as a consequence. Once the mood and/or anxiety disorder has been addressed, move on to targeted treatment of the OC spectrum disorder itself.

Forms of psychotherapy shown to be useful in adult patients with OC and related disorders are also generally believed to be useful for non-adults, although there are fewer rigorous trials. In all cases, psychotherapy will need to be modified so that it is age appropriate: consider use of language and communication styles, and whether any reinforcements and rewards are age-appropriate.

Disorder-specific psychological options for each condition are considered below:

- *Obsessive Compulsive Disorder.* CBT with Exposure and Ritual Prevention (ERP) is used in children and adolescents and has a reasonable evidence base. ERP is undertaken in a gradual fashion and requires a good understanding of the underlying OCD symptoms and a sensitive therapist skilled in communicating with young people. This process should include sessions involving parent(s) and the setting of age and development appropriate homework assignments. The use of positive reinforcements (e.g., small rewards from parents or the therapist) for progress can be helpful.
- *Hoarding Disorder.* There are only a few case reports examining psychological treatments specifically for childhood hoarding. In the absence of rigorous trials, we recommend that CBT with ERP be utilized, based on positive experiences in child OCD patients, including child OCD patients with hoarding symptoms.
- *Tic Disorders.* Childhood Tic Disorders are amongst the best studied in terms of psychological treatment options. The available evidence supports the use of habit reversal training (HRT), a short-term behavioral intervention that focuses on helping individuals to be more aware of their tics and to use competing responses (CRs). HRT was first established in the 1970s. The therapist typically begins by making a list of current tics from most bothersome to least bothersome, from the sufferer's perspective. Tics that have clear preceding feelings/urges and which lead to a simple "conditioned" response are most likely to be amenable to treatment, and one such is selected from the list to begin with. Children are then taught "awareness training" to recognize the onset of premonitory urges/feelings before the given tic; this includes homework in which the child spends time at home monitoring their tics for a defined period each day. Next, the therapist works with the child to develop

alternative responses to be undertaken during premonitory urges or when tics first initiate (competing response or CR). For example, one CR could be moving one's head to a midline position and then tilting the chin and head down. Essentially, the CR should be less noticeable than the tic and incompatible with the tic. For vocal tics, slow steady breathing can be a useful CR. Again, practice is needed at home. Parents can be included in the therapeutic process by encouraging children to make use of the technique and providing small rewards or reinforcements for good progress.

- *Trichotillomania* and *Excoriation (Skin Picking) Disorder.* Habit reversal training (HRT), described above for Tic Disorders, has a good evidence base in the treatment of Trichotillomania in children, albeit in a slightly different format. For awareness training, the individual focuses on acts that precede pulling, such as moving one's head to the side and moving one's arm towards the eyebrows. For competing responses, examples include clenching one's fist or placing hands under one's legs. Unlike in HRT for tics, an additional technique used for Trichotillomania is stimulus control: modifying the environment to reduce exposure to hair pulling-related cues. Again, parents can be enlisted to encourage children to use the techniques and reward good progress, and homework is integral to the treatment along with considering social aspects (encouragement of social engagement and hobbies). While not well studied, HRT is likely to be useful for Excoriation Disorder as well as for Trichotillomania.
- *Illness Anxiety Disorder (Hypochondriasis).* There are very few (if any) trials examining structured therapies for Hypochondriasis in children. In general terms, psychological treatment should focus on education, reinforcement, and coping skills. Education involves considering the link between psychological and physical states, both in terms of the child and in terms of dynamics between the child and wider family; including family members, especially parents, in therapy is critical. In terms of reinforcement, children

should be rewarded (both verbally by parents and also potentially with small physical rewards) for engaging in positive activities while possible "reinforcers" for maladaptive illness behavior should be identified and removed. Coping skills can include families spending time together on fun activities when the child presents as being relatively symptom free. Parents should be seen by the therapist both with the child and separately. Treatment is likely to be difficult for parents since it may entail ignoring certain behaviors despite considerable agitation on the part of the child, hence the need to provide them, as well as the child, with supportive input.

- *Body Dysmorphic Disorder.* CBT can be useful in the treatment of childhood Body Dysmorphic Disorder (BDD), provided it is appropriately tailored, and incorporates Exposure and Ritual Prevention (ERP). Such CBT can include making lists of the pros and cons of changing BDD behaviors to start with, along with making an "anxiety hierarchy" of BDD-related scenarios. The child can then work with the therapist on exposing themselves to these situations while not ritualizing, starting with the least anxiety-provoking situation. This would include homework assignments. Some studies have incorporated perceptual retraining, helping children to see their entire body when looking in mirrors, rather than honing in on specific details in a compulsive fashion. Parents can be enlisted in helping children with homework activities, and can give small rewards for positive results. CBT should also incorporate psychoeducation and encourage the use of distraction techniques, along with re-engagement with social and other enjoyable activities.

When considering drug treatments for pediatric OC spectrum disorders:

- Be sure to assess for suicidal thoughts and thoughts of self-harm at baseline and during treatment (there is some evidence that SSRIs can increase suicidal ideations in depressed non-adults, and this should be mentioned where relevant).

- Warn patients and their families that
  - Side effects are more common when treatment is first started. If side effects can be tolerated, they often settle down with time.
  - OC symptoms may get worse initially (over the first 1–2 weeks of treatment).
  - Beneficial effects take time to show themselves; for most OC spectrum disorders, medication at a therapeutic dose for 8–12 weeks is needed before deciding whether or not the treatment has led to benefits.
  - Monitoring is needed for some kinds of medication (e.g., with antipsychotic medication, which would require physicals, blood tests, and ECG/EKG).

Disorder-specific pharmacological options for pediatric OC spectrum disorders are summarized below in Table 10.1. You should also refer to the disorder-relevant chapter elsewhere in this book.

Key References

- Dutta N, Cavanna AE. The effectiveness of habit reversal therapy in the treatment of Tourette syndrome and other chronic tic disorders: a systematic review. Funct Neurol. 2013 Jan-Mar;28(1):7–12.
- Freeman J, Garcia A, Frank H, Benito K, Conelea C, Walther M, Edmunds J. Evidence-Base Update for Psychosocial Treatments for Pediatric Obsessive Compulsive Disorder. J Clin Child Adolesc Psychol. 2014;43(1):7–26.
- Hwang GC, Tillberg CS, Scahill L. Habit reversal training for children with tourette syndrome: update and review. J Child Adolesc Psychiatr Nurs. 2012 Nov;25(4):178–83.
- Masi G, Pfanner C, Brovedani P. Antipsychotic augmentation of selective serotonin reuptake inhibitors in resistant tic-related obsessive compulsive disorder in children and adolescents: a naturalistic comparative study. J Psychiatr Res. 2013 Aug;47(8):1007–12.

TABLE 10.1 Overview of Pharmacological Treatment Options for Childhood OC Disorders

Disorder	*Specific medication options*		
	Name	*Side effects*	*Age range and corresponding dosing recommendations*
Obsessive Compulsive Disorder	General Comments: There is evidence to support the use of SSRIs from controlled trials. No blood or EKG/ECG monitoring is needed with SSRIs listed here, unless there are specific cardiac concerns. Clomipramine is second-line, where one or more adequate courses of SSRI have failed. Clomipramine is superior to placebo in the treatment of children with OCD; baseline and follow-up EKGs/ECGs are recommended. Where available, clomipramine plasma levels should be monitored (hence avoid in children where needle phobia is present)		
	Sertraline	Nausea, headache, nervousness, sleep disturbance, and diarrhea	Aged 6–12 years: initially 25mg daily, increase to 50mg daily after one week, further increase in steps of 50mg/day at intervals of one week if needed. Maximum 200mg/day. Aged 12 years and above: initially 50mg daily, increased in steps of 50mg/day at intervals of at least one week if needed. Maximum 200mg/day

(continued)

TABLE 10.1 Continued

Disorder	*Specific medication options*		
	Name	***Side effects***	***Age range and corresponding dosing recommendations***
	Fluoxetine	As above	Aged 7 and above: 10mg daily increased by 10mg/day every 1–2 weeks if necessary and tolerated. Maximum 30mg/day
	Fluvoxamine	As above	Aged 8 and above: Initially 25mg daily, increase in steps of 25mg/day every 1 week as necessary. When total daily dose is over 50mg, give in divided doses. Maximum total daily dose 200mg
	Clomipramine	Dry mouth, tiredness, dizziness, tremor, headache, constipation, loss of appetite, abdominal discomfort, and insomnia	Aged 10 and above: Titrate to target a dose of 3mg per kg per day
Hoarding	General Comments: Limited evidence base. Treat as for childhood OCD		
Tic Disorders	General Comments: Clonidine and guanfacine are non-antipsychotic medications with moderate quality evidence in terms of efficacy; useful when treating Tic Disorder plus ADHD. Certain antipsychotic medications have excellent quality evidence in terms of efficacy but side effects can be problematic; there is the need for ECG/EKG and blood monitoring with antipsychotics		

	Clonidine	Sedation, bradycardia, orthostatic hypotension, and dry mouth. Risk of rebound syndrome if stopped suddenl.	Aged 7 and above: Titrate dose gradually according to blood pressure and heart rate—start at 0.025mg/day, increase over time to maximum 0.1mg/day. There is also a clonidine patch available: treatment dose is 1–2mg clonidine patch applied once per week. Patches can cause local skin irritation
	Guanfacine	Fatigue, headache, and sleep disturbance	Aged 7 and above: Titrate dose gradually according to blood pressure and heart rate—start at 0.5mg/day, increase over time to maximum 3mg/day
	Pimozide	Sedation, prolactin elevation, weight gain, hypercholesterolemia, QT prolongation, and extrapyramidal side effects (EPSEs)	Aged 12 and above: Titrate dose gradually starting at 1mg/day. Step up dose once weekly in 1mg/day increments. Maximum 4mg/day
	Haloperidol	As above	Aged 7 and above: Titrate dose gradually starting at 0.5mg three times/day (1.5mg total daily dose). Recommended maximum 1mg three times/day (3mg total daily dose). [EPSEs more likely with haloperidol versus the other options]

(continued)

TABLE 10.1 Continued

Disorder	*Specific medication options*		
	Name	*Side effects*	*Age range and corresponding dosing recommendations*
	Risperidone	As above	Aged 7 and above: Titrate dose gradually starting at 0.5mg/day, increasing in once weekly steps of 0.5mg/day. Maximum dose 1.5mg/day
Trichotillomania	General Comments: No pharmacological treatment can be recommended. There have been virtually no studies of pharmacotherapies in non-adult patients. Contrary to findings in adults, the one available blinded treatment trial using *n*-acetylcysteine (NAC) in children with Trichotillomania showed no significant benefit compared to placebo		
Skin Picking Disorder	General Comments: No pharmacological treatment can be recommended. There have been virtually no studies of pharmacotherapies in non-adult patients		
Illness Anxiety Disorder (Hypochondriasis)	General Comments: Little is known about pharmacological treatment of Hypochondriasis in non-adults. No pharmacological treatment can be recommended in general. Consider SSRIs for individuals approaching adult age (16–17 year olds)—see chapter 6 for options		
Body Dysmorphic Disorder (BDD)	General Comments: Little is known about pharmacological treatment of BDD in non-adults. No pharmacological treatment can be recommended in general. Consider SSRIs for individuals approaching adult age (16–17 year olds)—see chapter 5 for options		

- Phillips KA, Rogers J. Cognitive-behavioral therapy for youth with Body Dysmorphic Disorder: current status and future directions. Child Adolesc Psychiatr Clin N Am. 2011 Apr;20(2):287–304.
- Storch EA, Rahman O, Park JM, Reid J, Murphy TK, Lewin AB. Compulsive hoarding in children. J Clin Psychol. 2011 May;67(5):507–16.
- Weisman H, Qureshi IA, Leckman JF, Scahill L, Bloch MH. Systematic review: pharmacological treatment of tic disorders—efficacy of antipsychotic and alpha-2 adrenergic agonist agents. Neurosci Biobehav Rev. 2013 Jul;37(6):1162–71.

Alternative Treatments

The majority of published trials for OCD and Related Disorders have considered psychotherapy (notably CBT) and mainstream pharmacological agents such as serotonin reuptake inhibitors (e.g., clomipramine, fluoxetine). This chapter considers other potential interventions for OC and Related Disorders—the so-called alternative treatments—which have received far less attention to date.

In general, selection of treatment for any condition is dependent upon a balance between benefits (clinical efficacy) and costs (side effects, access, monetary costs, time costs). Ideally, aspects of benefits/costs would be evaluated in controlled clinical trials, meta-analyses, and systematic reviews. Treatment guidelines for most disorders have evaluated studies based on a hierarchy of quality of evidence, ranging from low-level evidence (as seen in case reports and uncontrolled studies) to top-level (multiple randomized controlled trials).

Although OCD has a large number of treatment studies supporting the guidelines, many of the related disorders lack definitive evidence regarding treatment approaches. This poverty of evidence is even more extreme in the context of alternative treatments, for which in many instances only case reports are available. In our view, if the alternative treatment lacks high quality evidence, they should not be used inlieu of more mainstream treatments; rather, they may have a role in complementing more validated treatments.

Who Are These Treatments For?

Research indicates that symptom improvement for OCD and Related Disorders often ranges from 30–60% when standard treatments (e.g., CBT, SRIs) are used, leaving the patient with remaining symptoms that could potentially be treated concurrently with other techniques. Several other situations may arise when alternative treatments should be considered:

1. Someone cannot tolerate usual medications (e.g. SRIs) or their side effects.
2. Someone could not undergo CBT or SRIs for financial reasons or because treatments are not available in their area.
3. Someone received inadequate or incomplete symptom improvement with SRIs or therapy.
4. Philosophically, someone is opposed to mainstream treatment.

Remember, these treatments can be used in conjunction with CBT and SRIs as augmentations. Most of the clinical trials for OCD and Related Disorders in which these interventions were implemented were done in conjunction with either CBT or SRIs. For patients who fall into one of the situations above, however, the following treatment options should be considered.

People should be cautioned that although many alternative treatments appear safe, they should always ask their doctors before starting any supplement. It is important that people do not mix chemicals, whether they are natural or synthetic or a combination, without a full and complete understanding of potential interactions. In addition, just because something might be appropriate in small doses does not mean that more is better or safe.

Possibly helpful alternative treatment options for the different OC conditions are summarized in Table 10.2, and are considered in more detail below.

Supplements/All-Natural Treatments

Note: these treatments are listed alphabetically rather than in order of preference

Borage (Echium amoenum)

Indications and Efficacy

Borage (Echium amoenum), is a dried flower used traditionally in the Persian culture as an anxiolytic and thymoleptic. The seed oil form of borage is generally the only version available in nutritional stores. At this time, we are unaware of any commercially available pill versions of borage with the flower extract. The flower and leaves, however, have been used to treat many conditions including fever, cough, depression, Attention Deficit Hyperactivity Disorder, and OCD. Documentation of borage use dates back to the Roman period of 300 BC.

The exact mechanism of borage in psychiatric illnesses is not clearly understood. The following use of borage in OCD is based upon use of the flower extract. The seed oil has not been studied.

Obsessive Compulsive Disorder. Borage (125mg capsules taken 1 capsule in the morning, 1 in the afternoon and 2 in the evening; capsules contained an aqueous extract made from borage flowers) was found to be effective in reducing obsessive and compulsive symptoms in 44 adult subjects randomly assigned to receive either borage extract or a matching placebo over a six-week period. In addition to reducing OCD symptoms, patients taking borage also benefited in terms of anxiety and depressive symptoms.

Initiation and Ongoing Treatment

The target dose of borage is not well established. Dosing between 375–500mg per day is a reasonable target.

Borage is available in oil form. For the flower extract (should a form be available), it should be prescribed at a maximum dose of 500mg per day. Pills should be given in 125mg per pill form.

TABLE 10.2 Possibly Helpful Alternative Treatments by Condition

Condition	*Supplements/ all-natural*	*Other treatments*
Body Dysmorphic Disorder	Glycine	Exercise
Excoriation (Skin Picking) Disorder	Inositol	Exercise, hypnosis
Trichotillomania	Inositol, n-acetylcysteine	Exercise, hypnosis, yoga
Hoarding Disorder		
Illness Anxiety Disorder (Hypochondriasis)		Acupuncture, exercise
Obsessive compulsive disorder	Borage, glycine, inositol, milk thistle, *n*-acetylcysteine, valerian root	Acupuncture, exercise, hypnosis, yoga
Tic disorders (Including Tourette's Syndrome)		Acupuncture, exercise, hypnosis

An example of a possible dose titration schedule for the flower extract is:

125mg by mouth in the morning (between 0800–0900)
125mg by mouth in the afternoon (between 1300–1500)
250mg by mouth at night (between 2100–2300)

Given the potential for liver damage with prolonged doses of borage, it should ideally only be prescribed for a maximum of one year, and monitoring of liver function via blood tests should be considered.

Risks and Side Effects

The most common side effects reported with borage treatment include headache and mild skin irritation (if the seed oil is used). The use of borage over a long period of time can irritate the liver, potentially causing liver damage and cancers. Patients should be advised to visit an emergency room for symptoms suggestive of anaphylactoid reactions.

Contraindications/Special Considerations

Pregnancy/breast-feeding. Borage may contain pyrrolizidine alkaloids which can cause liver damage, cancer, and birth defects as they may pass into the breast milk of the mother. As such, treatment with borage is contraindicated in this population.

Liver disease/hepatitis. Pyrrolizidine alkaloids may worsen liver conditions. Since borage may contain pyrrolizidine alkaloids, it is contraindicated for individuals with liver disease or hepatitis.

Bleeding disorders/surgical interventions. Borage seed oil might prolong bleeding time and increase the risk of bruising. As such, patients should be instructed to stop taking seed oil borage at least three weeks before a scheduled surgery in order to prevent potential complications from excess bleeding both pre- and post-surgery. Patients with a bleeding disorder should not take any version of borage.

Glycine

Indications and Efficacy

Glycine is an amino acid and is thought to act on N-methyl-D-aspartate (NMDA) receptors. Glycine has been examined in the treatment of a variety of medical conditions, including schizophrenia. Glycine is generally available in nutritional stores as a powder. The exact mechanism of glycine in psychiatric illnesses is not clearly understood.

Obsessive Compulsive Disorder. Glycine powder (30 grams twice a day) was found to be helpful in decreasing both obsessive and compulsive symptoms in a double-blind trial of 24 patients with OCD as adjunctive therapy to standard SRI pharmacotherapy. Compliance was a difficult issue in the study given participant complaints about taste and nausea associated with such high doses of glycine. At the end of the study, only 3 of the original 12 assigned to glycine had completed the study, limiting the interpretation of glycine efficacy in OCD.

Body Dysmorphic Disorder. One uncontrolled case report of a woman with both BDD and OCD, refractory of other treatments, found that glycine was effective in reducing both the OCD and BDD symptoms. The dose of glycine was 0.8 grams per kilogram per day.

Initiation and Ongoing Treatment

The target dose of glycine is not well established. Dosing between 40 and 60 grams per day is a reasonable target.

Glycine is available in a powder form and should be dissolved in either water or juice. It should be titrated to an optimal dose of 0.8g/kg of body weight. Dosing should be conducted in increments of 4g per day until this dose is reached and should be accomplished in within one and a half to three weeks. As such, the range of glycine dose will likely be titrated to a fixed daily dose of between 40g and 100g per day based upon body weight.

An example of a possible dose titration schedule is (e.g., 70 kilogram [155 lbs] man)

Day 1: 4 grams after breakfast each day (increase by 4 grams each day in divided doses)
Day 2: 4 grams in the morning after breakfast and 4 grams after dinner
Day 3: 8 grams in the morning after breakfast and 4 grams after dinner
Day 4: 8 grams in the morning after breakfast and 8 grams after dinner
Day 14: 28 grams in the morning after breakfast and 28 grams after dinner

Dosages should only be increased based on clinical severity and improvement as determined by the treating physician.

Risks and Side Effects

The most common side effects reported with glycine treatment include nausea, upset stomach, drowsiness, and vomiting. Patients should be advised to visit an emergency room for symptoms suggestive of anaphylactoid reactions.

Contraindications/Special Considerations

Pregnancy/breast-feeding. A limited amount of information is available regarding the use of glycine in pregnancy or breast-feeding women. As such, treatment with glycine is not recommended in this population.

Inositol

Indications and Efficacy

Inositol (or myo-inositol), a glucose isomer and second messenger precursor, is available in nutritional stores as a powder or a capsule (we recommend the powder only because it is easier to use and has been used in most of the treatment studies). The exact mechanism of inositol is not clearly understood. It has a slightly sweet taste and can be added to juice, cereal, yogurt, water, or any food item.

Obsessive Compulsive Disorder. Inositol has been shown to be effective in one placebo-controlled, double-blind trial of 13 patients with OCD. Inositol decreased OCD symptoms significantly more than placebo over a 6-week period. There is some indication, however, that inositol may be helpful in only a minority of OCD patients who add it to an SRI when they have inadequate response to the SRI.

Trichotillomania/Excoriation (Skin Picking) Disorder. In the case of these OCD-related disorders, there are no placebo-controlled double-blind data to support the use of inositol. In an open-label study, however, three women with Trichotillomania and Excoriation Disorder all improved when taking inositol.

Initiation and Ongoing Treatment

The target dose of inositol is 12–18 grams per day. It can be titrated to a maximum dose of 18 grams per day.

Dose changes should follow a systematic approach whereby dose titration should start at 2 grams three times a day (breakfast, lunch, dinner) and be increased over a period of a few weeks to 18 grams per day (6 grams 3 times a day) based on clinical assessment of improvement and adverse events.

An example of a possible dose titration schedule is:

(Note: Inositol: 1–1.5 teaspoon=2 grams)
Day 1: 1–1.5 teaspoon by mouth, three times per day
Day 7: 2–3 teaspoons by mouth, three times per day
Day 21: 3–4.5 teaspoons by mouth, three times per day

Dosages should only be increased based on clinical severity and improvement as determined by the treating physician.

Risks and Side Effects

Risks

Risks are minimal. Inositol is generally well-tolerated and appears to be safe for patients to take. Allergic reactions to inositol have been reported and may include itching, hives, rash, wheezing, difficulty breathing, or swelling in the mouth or throat. Patients should be advised to visit an emergency room for symptoms suggestive of anaphylactic reactions.

Side Effects

Side effects from inositol include nausea, headache, tiredness, and diarrhea.

Side effects are usually mild and short term.

Most side effects, if experienced, will occur during the first 1–2 weeks of treatment.

Contraindications/Special Considerations

Pregnancy/breast-feeding. A limited amount of information is available regarding the use of inositol in pregnancy or breast-feeding women. As such, treatment with inositol is not recommended in this population.

Bipolar Disorder and patients taking lithium. One case report found that a patient's mania worsened when taking inositol in excessive amounts. The problem is that the person was also taking excessive amounts of caffeine. There are other reports, however, in the scientific literature that inositol appears safe and beneficial in people with bipolar disorder.

There is also some mention in the popular press that lithium and inositol may have a dangerous interaction. The scientific literature, however, suggests that inositol appears safe in those taking lithium and may in fact help with some side effects of lithium.

Given the lack of scientific clarity on these topics, we recommend patients who are taking lithium or have bipolar disorder to discuss this with their physicians before starting inositol.

Milk Thistle (Silybum marianum)

Indications and Efficacy

Milk thistle, or silybum marianum, has been described in the literature for hundreds of years as an herbal remedy for a number of physical and mental ailments. Research indicates that it may have anti-cancer, anti-inflammatory, anti-diabetic, and anti-oxidant qualities and is used in many countries for liver disorders, including cirrhosis and hepatitis.

Milk thistle is generally available in nutritional stores as a capsule (in a variety of doses). The exact mechanism of milk thistle in psychiatric illnesses is not clearly understood, although the theory is that the flavanoid complex silymarin may increase serotonin levels in the cortex.

Obsessive Compulsive Disorder. Milk thistle demonstrated efficacy in one double-blind trial of 35 patients with moderate to severe OCD randomized to receive either milk thistle extract (in the form of a pill; 200mg by mouth three times per day) or fluoxetine (10mg by mouth three times per day. At the end of the trial, both treatment groups demonstrated significant symptom severity improvement.

Initiation and Ongoing Treatment

The target dose of milk thistle is 600mg per day.

Dose changes should follow a systematic approach whereby dose titration should start at 200mg a day (after a meal) and be increased over a period of a couple weeks to 600mg a day (200mg three times a day after each meal) based on clinical assessment of improvement and adverse events.

An example of a possible dose titration schedule is:

Day 1: 200mg by mouth after breakfast each day
Day 7: 200mg by mouth twice per day (after breakfast and dinner)
Day 14: 200mg by mouth three times per day (after each meal)

Dosages should only be increased based on clinical severity and improvement as determined by the treating physician.

Any benefit for OCD may require at least 5–6 weeks of treatment.

Risks and Side Effects

Risks

Milk thistle may cause an allergic reaction in people who are sensitive to the Asteraceae/Compositae plant family or to daisies, artichokes, common thistle, kiwi, or to any of milk thistle's constituents (silibinin, silychistin, silydianin, silymonin, siliandrin). Anaphylactic shock (a severe allergic reaction) from milk thistle tea or tablets has been reported in several patients. It should not be prescribed for individuals with an allergy to this family of plant.

Milk thistle may interact with different medications by reducing their breakdown in the liver and thereby increasing their serum levels. Medications metabolized by cytochrome P450 2C9 (e.g., phenytoin, tamoxifen, glipizide, warfarin, diazepam), cytochrome P450 3A4 (e.g., ketoconazole) or by glucuronidation (e.g., digoxin, estrogen, lamotrigine, morphine) may be affected by milk thistle. Before starting milk thistle, patients should talk with their physicians.

Side Effects

The most common side effects reported with milk thistle treatment include diarrhea, bloated feeling, nausea, and loss of appetite.

Contraindications/Special Considerations

Pregnancy/breast-feeding. A limited amount of information is available regarding the use of milk thistle in pregnancy or breast-feeding women. As such, treatment with milk thistle is not recommended in this population.

Breast cancer, ovarian cancer, or uterine cancer. In hormone-sensitive conditions such as these, milk thistle extract might act like estrogen. As such, for female patients in treatment or remission from cancer, milk thistle is contraindicated.

N-acetylcysteine (NAC)

Indications and Efficacy

Researchers have postulated that possible glutamatergic dysfunction may exist in patients with OCD and Related Disorders and have found that children with OCD may have reduced glutamatergic transmission in the anterior cingulate cortex.

N-acetylcysteine (NAC), a glutamatergic agent thought to attenuate glutamate transmission, has shown efficacy in treating a number of psychiatric and other medical disease states, including Trichotillomania in adults, excoriation (Skin Picking) Disorder, and onychophagia (pathological nail biting). It has been shown to decrease urges to engage in substance (nicotine, cocaine, cannabis) use and behavioral (gambling) disorders.

Obsessive Compulsive Disorder. NAC appears to be a potentially effective augmentation to SRI treatment in a double-blind trial of 48 adults with treatment-refractory OCD. The study found that a significantly higher proportion of the NAC-treated group experienced symptom reduction compared to the placebo group following 12-weeks of treatment.

Trichotillomania. Case reports and one double-blind trial of 50 adult patients with Trichotillomania demonstrated the efficacy of NAC in reducing the severity of hair pulling symptoms after 12 weeks of treatment. It is a recommended treatment for adult patients with Trichotillomania; however, NAC has not been shown to be beneficial in pediatric patients with Trichotillomania.

Excoriation (Skin Picking) Disorder. Limited data exist regarding the use of NAC in Excoriation Disorder. Case reports and case series suggest that NAC may be helpful in reducing the urges to pick and actual picking behaviors.

Initiation and Ongoing Treatment

Target dosing of NAC should be 1200mg–3000mg per day. Because it is a natural supplement available in grocery and vitamin stores made by many companies, the dose of the capsule may differ.

Dose changes should follow a systematic approach whereby dose titration should start at 1200mg per day (given as 600mg in divided doses) and be increased over a period of a few weeks to 3000mg per day (e.g., 1800mg in the morning and 1200mg in the evening) based on clinical assessment of improvement and adverse events.

An example of a possible dose titration schedule is:

Day 1: 600mg by mouth twice per day
Day 14: 1200mg by mouth twice per day
Day 28: 3000mg by mouth (1800mg by mouth each morning and 1200mg by mouth each evening)

The dose of NAC should not be increased if maximum improvement (per clinical judgment) is realized at a lower dose.

Following dose adjustments, if patients report side effects from NAC they should be instructed to drop the dose to the level at which they were pre-adjustment if the side effects are bothersome to the patient. For example, if a patient is titrated to 2400mg per day (1200mg by mouth, twice per day) and experiences an upset stomach, they should be instructed to drop the dose to 1200mg or 1800mg per day and see if the upset stomach continues. If symptoms worsen or continue to be bothersome to the patient, discontinuation of the medication is recommended.

Risks and Side Effects

Risks

Risks are minimal. NAC is well-tolerated and generally safe for patients to take. Many people recommend supplemental zinc, copper, and other trace minerals, as well as taking two to three times the typical amount of vitamin C. These recommendations are based on people taking NAC over "an extended period," and because the scientific literature is unclear as to what that actually means, it is probably best to take NAC with a multivitamin plus vitamin C.

Side Effects

Side effects from NAC include nausea, indigestion, headache, and abdominal pain. Side effects are usually mild and short term. They are generally seen in about 15% of people taking NAC.

Most side effects, if experienced, will be reported during the first 1–2 weeks of treatment. However, safety and tolerability should be monitored closely and appropriate interventions made. Patients should be advised to visit an emergency room for symptoms suggestive of anaphylactoid reactions.

Contraindications

Pregnancy/breast-feeding. A limited amount of information is available regarding the use of NAC in pregnancy or breast-feeding women. As such, treatment with NAC is not recommended in this population.

Asthma. Reports indicate that NAC may worsen asthma.

Valerian Root (Valeriana officinalis L)

Indications and Efficacy

Valerian is a flowering plant found in the northern hemisphere. It was primarily used in Persian culture and has been written about in the literature since the 16th century. It has numerous uses, including perfumes, sedation, as an anxiolytic, for pain relief, as an anticonvulsant, for insomnia, and migraines. Valerian contains aleuronic acid which is a modulator of $GABA_A$ receptors and isovaltrate, an agonist for adenosine A_1 receptor sites.

Valerian is found in many vitamin or health food stores where the extract of the root is sold in the form of capsules. It is generally touted as a treatment for insomnia.

Obsessive Compulsive Disorder. Valerian root appeared to be a potentially effective treatment in a double-blind trial of 31 adults with OCD. The study found that a significantly higher proportion of the valerian root-treated group experienced symptom reduction compared to the placebo group following 8-weeks of treatment. The study found that those taking valerian root separated significantly from placebo after 4 weeks of treatment.

Initiation and Ongoing Treatment

The study for OCD gradually increased doses over a few weeks and gave valerian throughout the day. Due to the sedating properties of valerian root, it may be wiser to take the total amount approximately 30 minutes before bed. The dose used in the OCD study was 750mg. For insomnia, valerian root is usually used anywhere from 400mg to 900mg each day.

Full treatment effect may not be realized until at least week 4 of treatment.

Risks and Side Effects

Side effects are generally mild in severity. The most common side effects reported with valerian root treatment include somnolence, insomnia, nausea, dry mouth, constipation, headache, and irritability. Patients should be advised to visit an emergency room for symptoms suggestive of anaphylactoid reactions.

Contraindications/Special Considerations

Pregnancy/breast-feeding. A limited amount of information is available regarding the use of valerian root in pregnancy or breast-feeding women. As such, treatment with valerian root is not recommended in this population.

Surgery. Valerian root has been known to depress the central nervous system. As such, individuals scheduled for surgical intervention should stop taking valerian root at least 3 weeks prior to surgery.

Other Treatments

Acupuncture

Acupuncture has been used in eastern medicine for hundreds of years, in a number of physical and mental health conditions. Among other effects, acupuncture has been shown to have analgesic and anti-inflammatory effects. Acupuncture may transiently affect a number of hormones in the central nervous system, including serotonin, noradrenaline, and beta-endorphins.

Obsessive Compulsive Disorder. Electroacupuncture has been shown to be effective in decreasing clinical severity scores when used in conjunction with ongoing SRI treatment in a wait-list control study. Patients with inadequate response to their SRI treatment were given 12 sessions of electroacupuncture (5 times per week) over a period of approximately two weeks. Subjects receiving the electroacupuncture treatment demonstrated significantly greater OCD symptom improvement compared to those in the wait-list control group.

Tourette's Syndrome. Acupuncture was shown to be beneficial in treating the symptoms of Tourette's Syndrome in a sample of 24 adults and in the treatment of hypochondriac pain. A larger sample of 156 children and adolescents with Tourette's Syndrome found that 92.3% of patients reported significant symptom reduction.

Trichotillomania. A study in which 44 women with Hair Pulling Disorder were interviewed about what they found to be effective treatments for their condition found that neither of the 2 patients who received acupuncture found it to be effective.

Initiation and Ongoing Treatment

Acupuncture should not be considered a stand-alone treatment for OCD. For OCD, acupuncture has only been shown to be effective in conjunction with recommended treatments such as SRIs or behavioral or cognitive therapies. In the case of Tourette's Syndrome, research suggests that children and adolescents may benefit significantly from acupuncture treatment. Acupuncture is not recommended for Trichotillomania. Acupuncture has been shown to be particularly effective in treating mood and anxiety symptoms and should be considered as an adjunctive treatment for patients presenting with co-occurring depression or anxiety. It should only be undertaken by trained practitioners who use standard equipment and sterile practices.

Risks and Side Effects

Minimal risks are associated with acupuncture treatment, when undertaken by trained practitioners. Irritation of the skin, mild bruising, or residual itching surrounding the site of needle application may occur. Other side effects may include mild nausea, dizziness, or light-headedness but should resolve shortly after the cessation of treatment.

Exercise

Moderate aerobic physical exercise has been shown to be effective in treating the symptoms associated with a variety of Obsessive Compulsive and Related Disorders, including two studies in OCD (11 adults treated over 6 weeks and 15 adults treated over 12 weeks), a case series of two children with Tourette's Disorder, and recommendations from the Mayo Clinic to help manage the symptoms of Body Dysmorphic Disorder or Hypochondriasis. Exercise can also be useful in treating the negative mood states and anxiety often associated with Trichotillomania and excoriation (Skin Picking) Disorder.

Indications and Efficacy

Aerobic exercise with moderate intensity coupled with behavioral therapy has been shown to be helpful in reducing the severity of OCD symptoms in a randomized clinical trial. Further trials assessing the effectiveness of exercise to improve OCD symptoms are ongoing.

Initiation and Ongoing Treatment

Exercise should not be considered a stand-alone treatment for OCD or related conditions. It has only been shown to be effective for OCD in conjunction with recommended treatments such as SRIs or behavioral or cognitive therapies.

Encouraging patients to engage in moderate aerobic exercise for at least 20–40 minutes 2–3 times per week is recommended but not as a first-line treatment for OCD or other body-focused repetitive behaviors.

Risks and Side Effects

There are minimal risks associated with encouraging patients to exercise, however, clinical judgment should be used for patients with a medical condition that puts the patient at higher risk for cardiovascular and/or respiratory complications.

Further, and since compulsive exercise may be a clinical symptom of conditions such as Body Dysmorphic Disorder or (conversely) avoidant in Hypochondriasis, it is vitally important that the clinician assess for the presence of exercise compulsivity or avoidance should the patient have BDD or Hypochondriasis.

Hypnosis

Indications and Efficacy

Hypnosis can include a wide array of techniques, including accessing the subconscious mind of the patient with OCD in order to better understand the underlying reasons behind the obsessions and compulsions and subsequently neutralize those unwanted thoughts and behaviors. Alternatively, it can be used to teach relaxation and meditation techniques.

Hypnosis has been shown to be useful in a sample of OCD patients, in case reports and case series for both children and adults with Trichotillomania or Tourette's Syndrome, and in a case report for the treatment of excoriation (Skin Picking) Disorder.

Initiation and Ongoing Treatment

Hypnosis should not be considered a stand-alone treatment for OCD, Trichotillomania, Tourette's Syndrome, or excoriation (Skin Picking) Disorder. Per NICE guidelines (UK), there is no clinically convincing evidence for the use of hypnosis as a viable treatment for OCD. Several Trichotillomania reports indicate that it may be considered a viable treatment, however, we recommend that it only be used for Trichotillomania if *n*-acetylcysteine or habit reversal therapy are either non-preferential to the patient or are contraindicated. In the case of Tourette's Syndrome, the use of hypnosis as an adjunctive treatment to habit reversal therapy, exposure and response prevention therapy, or pharmacotherapy, may be helpful in some patients.

Risks and Side Effects

There are minimal risks associated with hypnosis treatment. The most common side effect is a feeling of disorientation immediately following a hypnosis session. Patients who are actively abusing illicit substances or alcohol or who experience delusions or hallucinations should not undergo hypnosis.

Yoga

Indications and Efficacy

Kundalini yoga has been shown to be effective in treating OCD in a small, randomized trial of patients. Kundalini yoga involves meditative training, breathing exercises, chanting, and body awareness and flexibility. Patients who were treated over a period of three months with this form of yoga reported significantly greater OCD symptom improvement compared to a control group. Five of the patients in the trial also presented with Trichotillomania and showed symptom improvement in their hair pulling symptoms as well.

Initiation and Ongoing Treatment

Yoga should not be considered a stand-alone treatment for OCD or Trichotillomania. Limited data suggests that yoga is effective in treating OCD; however, we recommend that the clinician encourage the patient to use yoga techniques in conjunction with the use of

SRIs or behavioral or cognitive therapies. Yoga should also be considered an adjunctive treatment to *n*-acetylcysteine or habit reversal therapy in Trichotillomania.

If patients are interested in engaging in yoga, encourage him or her to contact a local health center or yoga club to inquire about courses that are available.

Risks and Side Effects

Minimal risks are associated with yoga, however, the clinician must assess for medical contraindications including cardiac complications prior to the recommendation of yoga.

Clinical Pearls for Alternative Treatments

- For OCD, alternative treatments should be considered as adjunctive to CBT or SRI therapy.
- *N*-acetylcysteine is an effective treatment for adults with Trichotillomania.
- Acupuncture, exercise, and yoga can be useful in improving mood and anxiety states for patients with OCD and related conditions, but should not be regarded as the first-line treatments.

Key References

- Sarris J, Camfield D, Berk M. Complementary medicine, self-help, and lifestyle interventions for obsessive compulsive disorder (OCD) and the OCD spectrum: a systematic review. J Affect Disord. 2012 May;138(3):213–21.

Hospitalization, Day Treatments, and Residential Treatments

Inpatient treatment and partial hospitalization programs have shown some benefit for patients with severe, treatment-refractory

OCD. These types of programs are only available at a few sites worldwide. For OC disorders apart from OCD, research is scant and tailored programs are even rarer.

Hospitalization

Hospitalization is largely called for when acute stabilization is needed. This may be the case for OCD patients with co-occurring depression who become suicidal or in the case of OCD patients who cannot manage any self-care (or food intake) due to the severity of their illness. Hospitalization is usually of short duration (i.e., a few days). In general, the types of therapies provided in most inpatient facilities do not directly treat OCD symptoms. As such, the patient will not be having their OCD directly addressed. For some, the OCD symptoms may actually worsen as they are prevented from engaging in compulsions but without the benefit of having therapist-directed lessons in cognitive restructuring.

Day Treatments/Partial Hospitalizations

Day treatment programs and partial hospitalization provide more intensive therapy services on an outpatient basis. The person may come to therapy a few days or every day of the week for a certain number of hours. Most programs deal with larger general issues of mood regulation and anxiety management. The majority of programs do not involve individualized therapy focusing on exposure ritual prevention that is needed for OCD.

Except in the case of day programs and partial programs specifically designed for OCD, the more general programs are often helpful for someone with co-occurring depression or anxiety who can function somewhat outside of an inpatient setting.

Intensive Residential Treatment (IRT)

An IRT program for OCD is appropriate in the case of severe OCD that is refractory to standard outpatient medication and cognitive behavioral treatments.

Although data are limited, some research indicates that IRT can be an effective treatment and that patients generally seem to improve by 30–50% on symptom and disability scores after undergoing IRT. Research also suggests that improvement seems to be maintained over time, after discharge from the program.

Some research further suggests that living alone after discharge is a significant predictor of worsening of OCD after completing such a program. Therefore, where possible, patients should be encouraged to engage with social support groups in order to reduce social isolation and enhance motivation.

How long is IRT? There is no set length for most programs but generally speaking the few available studies suggest that individuals with severe OCD might need approximately 2 months of treatment in an IRT for optimal results.

Day, Partial, and Residential Programs

What Type of Treatment Is Provided?

Most of these programs are multi-modal—combining careful physical, neurological, psychological, and social assessments with medication management, cognitive behavioral therapy, education about OCD, social skills deficits, interventions aimed at control issues, and family issues.

When Should These Types of Programs Be Considered?

- In the case of people who cannot comply with treatment—either because they are non-compliant with medications or because they cannot or will not undertake exposures on their own
- Those who have markedly impaired self-care or poor oral intake/dietary status
- Those whose OCD results in extreme or intolerable disruption to the home environment and family life

- The individual with co-occurring eating disorder, Substance Use Disorder, or severe mood disorder

Key References

- Boschen MJ, Drummond LM, Pillay A. Treatment of severe, treatment-refractory obsessive compulsive disorder: a study of inpatient and community treatment. CNS Spectr. 2008 Dec;13(12):1056–65.
- Boschen MJ, Drummond LM, Pillay A, Morton K. Predicting outcome of treatment for severe, treatment resistant OCD in inpatient and community settings. J Behav Ther Exp Psychiatry. 2010 Jun;41(2):90–5.

Neurosurgery for Obsessive Compulsive Disorder

Neurosurgery for psychiatric illness in the form of stereotactic ablation (selective destruction of brain tissue) dates back to the 1940s. Techniques initially developed in the context of treating movement disorders such as Parkinson's disease have more recently been applied to severe treatment-refractory OCD. Neurosurgery is sometimes used for severe treatment-refractory Tourette's Syndrome in adults, but due to a relative lack of controlled data, is not considered further here. There is no current role for neurosurgery for other OC family disorders in clinical practice, due to lack of trials/evidence, and so only OCD is considered further for the purposes of this section.

There has been considerable refinement in both stereotactic ablation methods and in the newer technique of deep brain stimulation (DBS). Contemporary ablation reproducibly places lesions in specific/focal brain targets, guided by magnetic resonance imaging (MRI), stereotactic instruments, and specialized software. Radiosurgery obviates the need for craniotomy. DBS does require craniotomy to implant stimulating electrodes in specific brain targets, but is intentionally non-ablative, and permits flexible and largely reversible modulation of brain function.

There is recognition that despite conscientious use of our best empirically based behavioral and medication treatments, some OCD patients continue to suffer severe symptoms and marked impairment. It is estimated that over 20% of OCD patients may be refractory to available psychological and pharmacological treatments.

Considerable clinical data support the effectiveness and safety of modern neurosurgery in the management of treatment-refractory severe OCD. In this context, psychiatric neurosurgery has consistently yielded substantial improvement in symptoms and functioning in 35–70% of cases, with morbidity and mortality drastically lower than earlier procedures.

Ethical Issues

Currently, neurosurgery is predominantly reserved for OCD patients with severe, incapacitating symptoms who have failed to improve adequately after aggressive use of behavioral and medication treatments.

Surgery is not recommended unless a multidisciplinary committee reaches consensus regarding its appropriateness for a given candidate and the patient gives informed consent.

Stereotactic Ablation

The three main anatomical lesion sites for treatment of OCD are indicated in the Figure 10.1. In each procedure, bilateral lesions are made stereotactically under MRI-guidance.

1. Anterior Cingulotomy

The lesion target for an anterior cingulotomy is within the anterior cingulate cortex (Brodmann areas 24 and 32) at the margin of the cingulum white matter bundle. This brain region is involved in action monitoring.

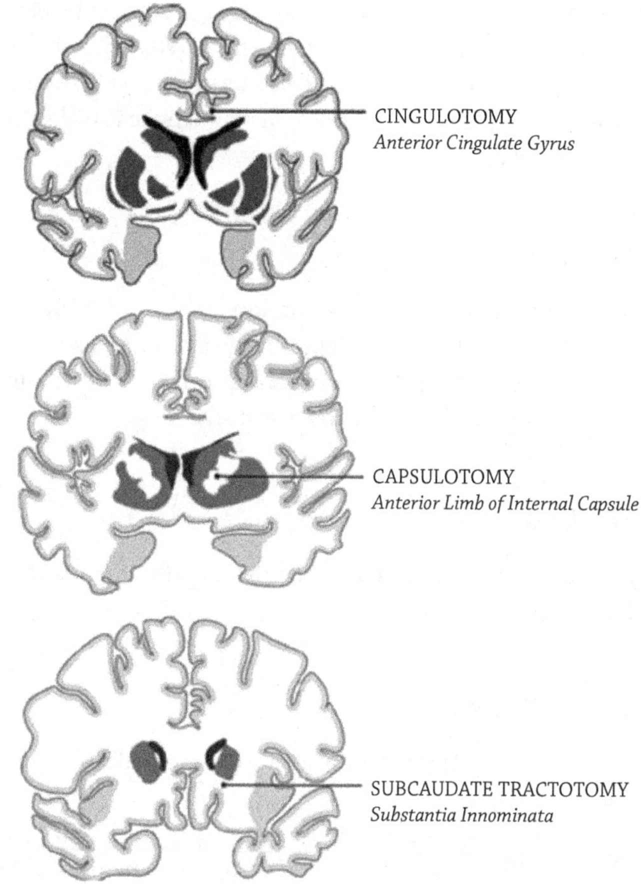

FIGURE 10.1 Key anatomical lesion sites for psychosurgical treatment of OCD. Reprinted with permission from Lipsman N, Neimat JS, Lozano AM: Deep Brain stimulation for treatment-refractory obsessive compulsive disorder: the search for a valid target. *Neurosurgery*. 2007; 61:1–13.

2. Capsulotomy

Anterior capsulotomy involves making lesions within the anterior limb of the internal capsule, impinging on the ventral stratum (part of the brain "reward system" which is likely to be involved in repetitive habits) immediately inferior to the capsule.

The intent is to interrupt fibers of passage between prefrontal cortex and subcortical nuclei including the dorsomedial thalamus. For over 15 years, capsulotomy has also been performed using the Leksell Gamma Knife, a radiosurgical instrument that makes craniotomy unnecessary.

3. Subcaudate Tractotomy

This procedure targets the substantia innominata (just inferior to the head of the caudate nucleus) with the goal of interrupting white matter tracts connecting the orbitofrontal cortex (involved in the generation of compulsions) to subcortical structures.

4. Limbic Leukotomy

Limbic leukotomy combines subcaudate tractotomy and anterior cingulotomy (1+3).

Outcomes after Ablation

Of these modern ablative procedures, anterior capsulotomy appears to be the most effective.

The literature suggests that approximately 60% of OCD patients had a therapeutic response (35% YBOCS improvement) to ablative procedures. It may take as long as 3–6 months for the beneficial effects to emerge. Potential side effects include headache, confusion, incontinence, weight gain, fatigue, memory loss, and seizure. Cingulotomies have a relatively low rate of side effects.

Deep Brain Stimulation

Deep brain stimulation (DBS) for psychiatric illness was tried as early as 1948 when JL Pool used stimulation through an electrode in the caudate nucleus in an attempt to treat a woman with depression and anorexia. In 2009, the American Food and Drug Administration (FDA) approved DBS in OCD even with little data, due to the recognition of the humanitarian need to treat severe OCD refractive to other treatments.

The current OCD DBS procedure is essentially the same as for routine use of DBS for movement disorders. Craniotomy is undertaken under local anesthesia, and patients are typically partially sedated but conscious during surgery. Lead placement, which is typically bilateral, is guided by multimodal imaging and specialized computerized targeting platforms. The most common targets for the placement of the leads are indicated in the Figure 10.2.

Outcomes for DBS: the overall response rate appears to exceed 50% in OCD for some DBS targets.

Side effects include hemorrhage, seizure, superficial infection, worsening of symptoms when DBS is stopped (e.g., due to battery failure), and transient hypomanic symptoms.

If Surgery Is Warranted, and Ethical Issues Have Been Addressed, Should Someone Choose Ablative Surgery or DBS?

The success rates for both ablative surgery and for DBS appear to be comparable but no direct comparisons studies have been conducted.

The main clinical advantages of DBS over lesion procedures are reversibility and adjustability. If DBS treatment is unsuccessful, the hardware can be explanted with little consequence for the patient. The available data from postmortem examination of brains from patients with implanted electrodes suggest that the pathological changes produced by chronic DBS are limited to minimal gliosis along the electrode tract.

One main disadvantage of DBS compared to radiosurgery is its relatively high cost (~$80,000 versus ~$15,000).

Certain centers around the world have experience with neurosurgical procedures for OCD.

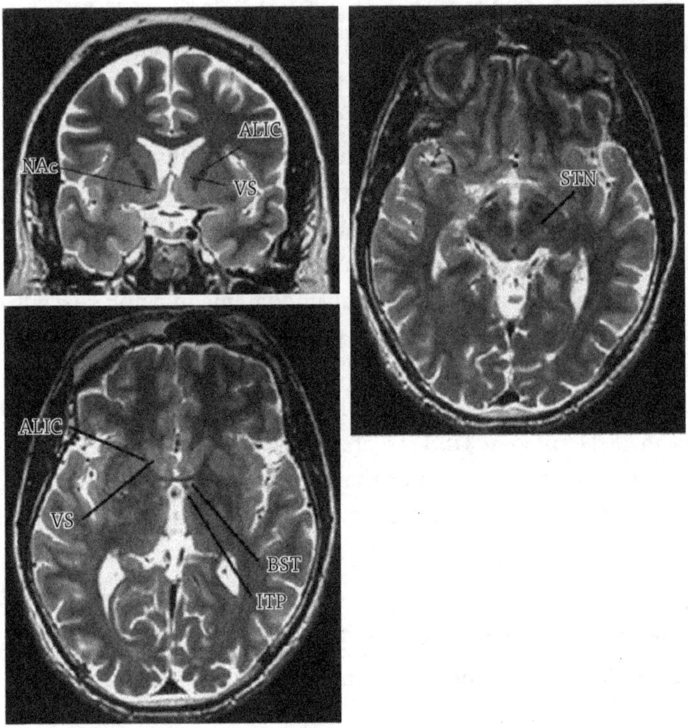

FIGURE 10.2 Main targets for DBS in OCD. NAc = nucleus accumbens, ALIC = anterior limb of the internal capsule, VS = ventral striatum, STN = subthalamic nucleus, BST = bed nucleus of the stria terminalis, ITP = inferior thalamic peduncle. Reprinted with permission from de Koning PP, Figee M, van den Munckhof P, Schuurman PR, Denys D. Current status of deep brain stimulation for obsessive compulsive disorder: a clinical review of different targets. Curr Psychiatry Rep. 2011 Aug;13(4):274–82.

Key References

- de Koning PP, Figee M, van den Munckhof P, Schuurman PR, Denys D. Current status of deep brain stimulation for obsessive compulsive disorder: a clinical review of different targets. Curr Psychiatry Rep. 2011 Aug;13(4):274–82.

- Figee M, Wielaard I, Mazaheri A, Denys D. Neurosurgical targets for compulsivity: what can we learn from acquired brain lesions. Neurosci Biobehav Rev. 2013 Mar;37(3):328–39.
- Greenberg BD, Rauch SL, Haber SN. Invasive circuitry-based neurotherapeutics: stereotactic ablation and deep brain stimulation for OCD. Neuropsychopharmacology. 2010 Jan;35(1):317–36.

11

Special Clinical Circumstances

Obsessive Compulsive Disorder and Substance Addiction

Although research on OCD has improved treatment for individuals suffering from this disorder, relatively little attention has been paid to the influence of Substance Use Disorders (abuse and/or dependence) in this population and how best to treat individuals when both disorders co-occur. Among individuals with OCD, approximately 25% have a lifetime Substance Use Disorder (23.2% with a lifetime alcohol use disorder and 13.3% with a lifetime drug use disorder).

Rates of Substance Use Disorders are even higher among patients with Body Dysmorphic Disorder (BDD) than the rates found in OCD. Around 50% of people with BDD have a lifetime history of one or more Substance Use Disorders, and current Substance Use Disorders are likely to be present in approximately 20% of BDD patients.

Among individuals with OCD, approximately three-quarters (77%) report onset of OCD prior to developing the substance addiction. Therefore, OCD may also be a precipitating factor in the development of substance addiction.

The substances most often abused by OCD subjects are alcohol and cannabis, which patients can perceive as being capable of temporarily 'relieving their anxiety' or as a means of 'getting away' from symptoms and their consequences. Clinicians should emphasize to patients that while such substances may provide transient relief, in the long-term there is evidence that they can make mental health worse and even interfere with treatment success.

Clinical Aspects of Co-morbid Substance Addiction

Patients with OCD and substance addiction generally have more severe OCD symptoms, poorer insight into OCD symptoms, poorer quality of life, and worse overall functioning. They are also more likely to be receiving disability allowances. Individuals with OCD or BDD and a substance addiction are at greater risk for suicide attempts and psychiatric hospitalizations than such individuals without a Substance Use Disorder.

OCD patients with substance addiction are more likely to have co-morbid personality disorders (especially Obsessive Compulsive Personality and Borderline Personality Disorders).

Recognizing co-morbidity with substance addictions in OCD is important, as identifying and treating the substance addiction is likely to significantly improve the prognosis.

This may be particularly important in individuals with OCD, given that certain psychoactive substances, such as cocaine or methamphetamine, may exacerbate obsessional symptoms, whereas other substances, such as opiates, may be enticing for patients because they may potentially alleviate obsessional symptoms.

Screening OCD Patients for Substance Addictions

All patients should undergo a screen for substances of abuse. Asking patients about what alleviates or worsens their OCD is a starting point. If alcohol and drugs are part of their answer to that question, follow-up questions to establish frequency of use and whether use is problematic (i.e., interferes with functioning) are needed.

Urine toxicology testing is a useful, easy, and quick way to screen for many drugs of abuse. Also, if certain drugs are found on testing (amphetamine/methamphetamine, cocaine), many times the OCD may be improved by informing the patient that abstinence from these drugs can ameliorate the severity of the OCD symptoms.

If opiates are being used, the patient may not want to stop use if they find some benefit for their OCD. In that case, education needs to be provided to let the patient know that other options may benefit him but without the addictive potential and other health, legal, and social problems of illicit opiates.

Screening Patients with Substance Addiction for OCD

Substance addiction in OCD patients is often an unplanned consequence of untreated OCD, therefore when patients present with Substance Use Disorders, be careful to screen for OCD. Because certain psychoactive substances, such as opiates or marijuana, may be enticing for individuals with OCD as they may potentially alleviate obsessional symptoms, patients with OCD may develop an addiction to opiates or marijuana.

When a substance addiction is recognized, many clinicians fail to screen for OCD assuming that the addiction is the primary problem. Treatment of the substance addiction may result in continued relapse, however, until the underlying OCD is addressed. Screening all substance addicted patients for OCD, therefore, is necessary to help the OCD as well as the substance addiction.

Treatment

There are no data regarding whether to treat the substance addiction or OCD first or to treat both simultaneously. Effective treatment for OCD may differ substantially from treatment for a substance addiction. Although different treatments are involved, in our clinical experience with patients with OCD and substance addictions, we recommend that both conditions be treated simultaneously.

Medication Options

It is well established that the pharmacological first-line treatment of choice for OCD is a serotonin reuptake inhibitor (SRI) (for example, clomipramine, fluvoxamine, fluoxetine).

The data regarding the efficacy of SRIs in the treatment of addiction are largely unimpressive except when targeting co-occurring disorders or symptoms.

A range of treatment modalities are available for substance abusers and different modalities are appropriate at different phases of recovery.

Detoxification is the first phase of recovery and medications are often required to reduce symptoms of withdrawal. Longer acting benzodiazepines are typically used in alcohol withdrawal. Opioid withdrawal can be effectively managed using methadone, clonidine, naltrexone, or buprenorphine; specialist input is advised.

The second phase of recovery is active treatment provided in settings ranging from weekly outpatient counseling to ambulatory day programs to residential treatment. The content of these treatments tends to be multimodal, often using a disease or twelve step orientation supplemented with cognitive and behavioral strategies. Naltrexone, acamprosate, and disulfiram are medications approved by the Food and Drug Administration (FDA) (and agencies in countries besides the United States) for treating alcohol dependent patients. Ondansetron has been shown to be effective in treating early-onset (predominantly male) alcoholism.

Methadone, naltrexone, and buprenorphine are pharmacological options for maintenance treatment of opioid dependence.

A variety of medications have been evaluated for cocaine dependence, and *n*-acetylcysteine, disulfiram, and baclofen have demonstrated early promise in randomized controlled trials. These medications can generally be used safely with SRIs when treating substance addictions in OCD patients (except possibly fluvoxamine when used in methadone patients due to causing increased levels of methadone and potential toxicity).

N-acetylcysteine has also shown benefit for the treatment of cannabis dependence. There are limited data supporting effective medications for the treatment of anxiolytic and sedative, hallucinogens and other stimulant dependence.

Recommendations

For the OCD patient with alcohol addiction, naltrexone plus an SRI may be a useful combination as some evidence suggests naltrexone helps with cognitive inflexibility, a deficit that is likely to contribute to perseverative behaviors in OCD.

For OCD patients with cocaine or marijuana addiction, the addition of *n*-acetylcysteine to an SRI may be helpful as there is growing evidence that this type of agent (a glutamate modulator) may help with OCD as well.

The third phase of recovery is the maintenance phase. For some individuals, highly structured environments, such as halfway houses, are helpful in promoting long-term success. These structured living situations should be recommended cautiously, however, in the case of OCD patients who may find that these environments trigger and worsen OCD (e.g., living with many people with HIV or hepatitis C in a person with OCD contamination obsessions). These living situations may worsen OCD and thereby lead to relapse.

For others, some type of ongoing focus on recovery is important in the maintenance phase. Although the exposure ritual prevention therapy (ERP) form of cognitive behavioral therapy has shown clear benefit for OCD, when a substance addiction co-occurs with OCD, the therapy may also need to focus on relapse prevention forms of cognitive behavioral therapy. Attendance at twelve step programs such as Alcoholics Anonymous, Narcotic Anonymous, and Cocaine Anonymous is associated with better outcomes in numerous correlational studies. Alternative mutual support groups with less focus on the spiritual aspect of recovery, such as Women for Sobriety, SMART Recovery, and Rational Recovery are increasingly available across North America, with similar/equivalent groups available in other countries. These interventions can be used simultaneously with ERP for OCD.

Key References

- Blom RM, Koeter M, van den Brink W, de Graaf R, Ten Have M, Denys D. Co-occurrence of obsessive compulsive disorder and substance use disorder in the general population. Addiction. 2011 Dec;106(12):2178–85.

- Fontenelle LF, Oostermeijer S, Harrison BJ, Pantelis C, Yücel M. Obsessive compulsive disorder, impulse control disorders and drug addiction: common features and potential treatments. Drugs. 2011 May 7;71(7):827–40.
- Gentil AF, de Mathis MA, Torresan RC, Diniz JB, Alvarenga P, do Rosário MC, Cordioli AV, Torres AR, Miguel EC. Alcohol use disorders in patients with obsessive compulsive disorder: the importance of appropriate dual-diagnosis. Drug Alcohol Depend. 2009 Feb 1;100(1-2):173–7.
- Mancebo MC, Grant JE, Pinto A, Eisen JL, Rasmussen SA. Substance use disorders in an obsessive compulsive disorder clinical sample. J Anxiety Disord. 2009 May;23(4):429–35.

Obsessive Compulsive Symptoms in Developmentally Disabled Individuals

Overview

Obsessions, compulsions and rituals are frequently associated with intellectual or developmental disabilities (IDD) and autism. The obsessive compulsive behaviors occur at high rates among persons of all ages with developmental disabilities. In addition, IDD and autism frequently overlap, and the overlap is associated with an even greater risk for developing obsessions and compulsions.

Although OCD appears to be rare in persons with IDD (3.5%), obsessive, compulsive, and ritualistic symptoms are common. High rates of obsessive compulsive behaviors have been consistently reported in individuals with Prader-Willi Syndrome, and Down Syndrome has been associated with the unique form of OCD characterized as obsessional slowness (i.e., individuals spend several hours each day performing tasks of daily living which should be completed much quicker).

A potential link between sensory hypersensitivity and the use of excessive rituals may underlie these behaviors. Sensory processing refers to the way in which the nervous system manages incoming sensory information. Sensory dysfunction in a child is likely to be experienced as psychologically distressing and upsetting. Consequentially, the child may search for ways to calm themselves and thereby develop excessive ritualistic behavior. These ritualistic behaviors may also include OC-related activities such as hair pulling or compulsive skin picking, for which the clinician should assess.

Further, intellectual or developmental disabilities in obsessive compulsive related disorders, such as Trichotillomania, skin picking, and Tourette's Disorder or tics, can present challenges in diagnosis and treatment. These disorders are quite common in the mentally handicapped population as well. A study of 259 patients with mental retardation found that 5% exhibited symptoms of Trichotillomania and 16.6% had some form of motor and/or vocal tic. Further, skin picking is very commonly found in Prader-Willi syndrome (e.g., from 82% to 95% of clinical samples have been found to have significant skin picking), a neurodevelopmental disorder resulting in intellectual disabilities resultant from an abnormality at chromosome 15.

Diagnosis

A significant overlap in symptoms often occurs between OCD and those with an IDD, including repetitive behaviors and obsessional thinking. In such cases, making a proper diagnosis can become complicated, especially in milder cases.

Intellectual Disability (Intellectual Developmental Disorder [IDD])

Intellectual disability (intellectual developmental disorder) is a disorder initiating during the developmental period and that includes both intellectual and adaptive functioning deficits in conceptual, social, and practical domains. According to the DSM-5, the three criteria can be summarized as follows:

- Intellectual impairment must be confirmed by a formal assessment with a clinician incorporating relevant tests (deficits may include problem solving, thinking abstractly, judgment, reasoning, learning through experience, and in terms of academic learning).
- Adaptive functioning problems must be evident, which limit the ability of the individual to fulfill societal standards of self-care and responsibility (in the absence of support/external intervention).
- The onset of these difficulties occurs during the developmental period.

Screening Patients with a Developmental Disability for Obsessive Compulsive Symptoms

Areas of particular impairment in individuals with IDD include:

- Social communication deficits
- Behavioral and cognitive inflexibility
- Deficits in judgment and social awareness

When assessing obsessive compulsive symptoms in this population, the following guidelines may be useful:

They may not to be able to identify obsessions.
The potential lack of abstract thinking or ability to articulate his or her thoughts may limit the individual in identifying obsessions.
If obsessive thoughts are recognized, the person may not be able to assess their irrational quality.
Children or adults with IDD often exhibit problems in abstract reasoning skills, and are therefore unlikely to be aware that their obsessions and compulsions are excessive.
Compulsions may be the key component in diagnosis.

> Obsessive compulsive symptoms may manifest in the form of repetitive behaviors. Clinicians may be looking for classic compulsions such as counting, checking, or washing. If the individual lacks abstract reasoning skills, these may not be the presenting compulsions. Instead, compulsions exhibit as overdrinking, pacing, compulsive masturbation, etc.

For severe IDD individuals who present for treatment of obsessive compulsive behaviors, aggression may be a central concern of the caregiver. In such cases, it is important to assess when the aggressive outbursts typically occur or *only* occur when the individual is *prevented* from engaging in a certain behavior.

Scales

Individuals with IDD may have limited language skills and this in turn may make it difficult to directly interview the person or have the person complete forms. Knowledgeable informants may be necessary to use these measures.

The Compulsive Behavior Checklist for Clients with Mental Retardation (CBC) can be used to compile information regarding obsessive compulsive symptoms. The CBC includes five categories of various compulsions: ordering, completeness, checking and touching, cleaning, and grooming compulsions. It is a particularly useful tool in assessing the number of compulsions. The CBC is scored by adding the total number of compulsions or the number of categories endorsed.

Obsessive Speech Checklist (OSC) for Clients with Mental Retardation can be used to collect information on obsessive speech patterns in individuals with IDD. It should not be used for individuals with profound intellectual disabilities or who speak only with single words or short phrases. In addition, the OSC should be used in conjunction with the Compulsive Behavior Checklist.

Differential Diagnosis

Normal development: Repetitive, rule-governed, and inflexible behaviors in children are often referred to as *rituals*. Up to a certain degree, childhood rituals are considered normative in any child's development. Learning to focus one's attention and engaging in repetitive behaviors helps the child to achieve a sense of control and mastery of her sensory universe. Some children, however, may engage in an exaggerated amount of rituals, upsetting the daily routine and causing problems in their daily functioning. In pre-school age children, a high degree of childhood rituals have been shown to be related to increased anxiety and fears.

Stereotypic Movement Disorder (SMD). Stereotypic Movement Disorder (SMD) involves repetitive engagement in motor activities, including head banging or nodding, body rocking, self-biting, and hand waving that begin in the early developmental period. These behaviors are much more common in IDD individuals, although the repetitive—often compulsive—engagement in these behaviors may be misconstrued as the compulsions noted in OCD. Stereotypic Movement Disorders, however, are differentiated from obsessive compulsive symptoms in that they are fixed, localized, and are purposeless (i.e., they are not done in response to an obsessional thought). Similarly, in Hair Pulling Disorder and excoriation (Skin Picking) Disorder, the behavior may be driven by an urge and, furthermore, generally have a purpose. Ask the patient or family member: "What types of compulsive behaviors does the patient engage in regularly? Do the behaviors solely involve actions like head banging or nodding, body rocking, self-biting, hand waving, or something similar?"

Anxiety disorders. The link between childhood rituals and anxiety may be reflected in rituals involving excessive insistence that things be done "just so," rigid repetitiveness, and sensitivity to minute details (e.g., stains, defects), need for symmetry and exactness, and repeating rituals and counting compulsions.

Severe *hoarding behaviors* affect 16.4% of individuals with IDD. It may be important to regularly assess patients with IDDs for hoarding behaviors. Hoarding in children with IDD may represent genuine complex hoarding behaviors and may be amenable to cognitive-behavioral interventions.

Treatment

Pharmacotherapy

In a systematic literature review of clinical trials of clomipramine and SSRIs in the treatment of obsessive compulsive symptoms in IDD, the majority found improvements in global functioning and reductions in anxiety and repetitive and/or compulsive behaviors.

In particular, clomipramine may be an effective drug for reducing repetitive thoughts and actions and aggressive behavior and for improving some elements of social behavior, such as eye contact and verbal responsivity in adults with IDD.

Therefore, a typical course of clomipramine or an SSRI treatment is recommended; however, close monitoring of pill compliance and of behavioral response to the medication by a caregiver or family member is necessary. The caregiver or family member of the patient should use appropriate symptom monitoring logs or scales (such as the CBC) to collect and report progress or regression of the patient to the clinician.

Psychotherapy

Learning-based procedures subsumed under the term *behavior therapy* have been a hallmark for treating rituals. In addition, enhancing prosocial skills may help to offset or replace problem behaviors. A broad array of skills have been addressed in this regard such as working memory, attention to task, communication, physical activity, social skills, academic tasks, and domestic skills. Sensory extinction has also been used for repetitive behaviors. By eliminating the sensory reinforcing aspects of the activity and substituting another preferred, more appropriate sensory reinforcer, the ritual may decrease.

Research also indicates that targeting the underlying anxiety of the individual is effective in reducing compulsions and aggression for IDD individuals with obsessive compulsive symptoms.

If intellectually able, help the patient to understand their disorder and the expression of the obsessive compulsive symptoms.

Tailor interventions to fit with the surroundings of the patient. For example, if the patient's home environment is a group home or other supervised facility, the therapy should be focused on managing and changing the adverse behavior in that specific setting.

In most cases of IDD, it is also important to educate the family on how to manage obsessive compulsive symptoms and prevent complications. Providing the family or caregiver a means of contacting your office with questions following the appointment is vital.

Remember that when addressing the patient, talk directly to him or her and not the caregiver or family member that may be in the room.

Other Conditions

Trichotillomania. Traditional treatments for Trichotillomania, including habit reversal therapy, are difficult to implement given intellectual barriers. The use of overcorrection techniques (e.g., contingent on hair pulling, the patient is instructed to brush his or her hair for 10 minutes) or placing mittens on the hands of the patient to prevent pulling, have been shown to be effective in case studies of children and adults with mental retardation and Trichotillomania. These treatments should be considered with caution, however, as they are all subjective forms of punishment to the patient.

Skin picking in Prader-Willi syndrome. Skin picking is extremely common in Prader-Willi syndrome, a disorder characterized by mild to moderate mental retardation. Various medications have been shown to be helpful in reducing skin picking in case reports or small samples of patients with Prader-Willi syndrome, including topiramate, a combination of naltrexone and fluoxetine, and sertraline. Controlled studies of therapy for skin picking in Prader-Willi syndrome are lacking and first-line treatments such as habit reversal therapy or acceptance and commitment therapy may be too cognitively intensive for the patient but should be considered as first-line treatments in this population as well should the patient be able to participate. The use of topical antibiotics and the bandaging of excoriated sites is necessary for the health of the patient.

Treatment Choice and Sequencing of Treatment

Behavior therapy is the treatment of choice for this patient population. The use of SRI treatment is also recommended in conjunction with behavior therapy. Obtaining information from the family member or caregiver on outcomes that are important to them is also recommended.

Clinical Pearls for OCD in Developmentally Disabled Individuals

- Behavior therapy in conjunction with an SRI is the treatment of choice.
- If aggression is of concern to the clinician, the use of divalproex or carbamazepine can be considered.
- Must consider differential diagnosis of Stereotypic Movement Disorder.
- Compulsions may comprise the key component to the diagnosis of OCD in this population since individuals are often unable to clearly verbalize underlying obsessions.
- Where possible, involve the family and/or caregiver of the patient in collecting an accurate patient history and in treatment planning.

Key References

- Chadwick O, Kusel Y, Cuddy M, Taylor E. Psychiatric diagnoses and behaviour problems from childhood to early adolescence in young people with severe intellectual disabilities. Psychol Med. 2005 May;35(5):751–60.
- Clarke DJ. Psychopharmacology of severe self-injury associated with learning disabilities. Br J Psychiatry. 1998 May;172:389–94.
- Singer HS. Stereotypic movement disorders. Handb Clin Neurol. 2011;100:631–9.

Obsessive Compulsive Disorder with Poor Insight

OCD can present in a way that the clinician believes the person has a psychotic disorder. This can be particularly the case in individuals who have OCD with poor insight, which is defined as a relative lack of understanding of the degree to which one's obsessions and compulsions are unreasonable or excessive.

Individuals with OCD vary in the degree of insight they have about the accuracy of the beliefs that underlie their OCD symptoms. Many individuals have good or fair insight (e.g., the individual believes that the house definitely will not, probably will not, or may or may not burn down if the stove is not checked 30 times). Some have poor insight (e.g., the individual believes that the house will probably burn down if the stove is not checked 30 times), and a few (4% or less) have absent insight/delusional beliefs (e.g., the individual is convinced that the house will burn down if the stove is not checked 30 times). Insight can vary within an individual over the course of the illness.

The subtyping of OCD has been expanded for DSM-5 to allow clinicians to make a more detailed assessment of the individual and his or her disorder. Instead of the single specifier "with poor insight," as in DSM-IV-TR, DSM-5 includes a range of insight specifiers (good or fair, poor, absent). Because insight may fluctuate over time, the insight specifier has been changed to refer to the current presentation. The revised specifiers have the potential advantage of conveying the broad range of insight that can characterize OCD beliefs, including delusional beliefs.

How Does This Differ from Delusions?

Insight was the original feature distinguishing OCD from psychosis. OCD therefore must be carefully differentiated from psychotic disorders. Some individuals with OCD have poor insight or even delusional OCD beliefs. However, they have obsessions and compulsions (distinguishing their condition from delusional disorder) and do not have other features of schizophrenia or schizoaffective disorder (e.g., hallucinations or formal thought disorder).

How to Assess Insight?

Insight exists along a continuum from excellent to extremely poor. The Brown Assessment of Beliefs Scale (BABS) allows the clinician to examine the degree of insight. It is particularly useful for OCD but can also be used for other OC family conditions including Body Dysmorphic Disorder (BDD) and Hypochondriasis. The BABS is a 7-item clinician administered interview. Scores for each item range from 0 (non-delusional) to 4 (delusional).

Why Care about Insight?

15–36% of OCD patients have little or no insight. Lack of insight is correlated with more severe OCD symptoms, and difficulties with treatment compliance. OCD patients with poor insight are more likely to have depression and may have increased rates of schizotypal personal disorder.

Poor insight has been associated with obsessions focusing on responsibility for harm, religious concerns, and somatic issues. Patients with Hypochondriasis and BDD generally show poorer insight than people with OCD.

Treatment of Poor Insight?

Pharmacologic Treatment

Degree of insight may or may not influence a person's response to an SRI. Many people with poor insight respond well to SRIs when they are willing to take medication. Having said that, poor insight may best predict which patients will be reluctant to commence treatment and those who may be non-compliant.

People with poor insight have an equivalent response to pharmacologic treatment regardless of the SRI agent being used.

There is no evidence that the addition of an antipsychotic is useful for poor insight OCD as first-line intervention, although antipsychotics are a potentially beneficial augmentation strategy for treatment-resistant OCD, this seems to be independent of whether or not the person has poor insight.

Psychotherapy Treatment

Can Exposure and Response Prevention (ERP) be used with poor insight OCD?

Patients with extremely poor insight show a poorer response to ERP. Patients with moderately or mildly poor insight can respond to ERP.

Poor insight OCD patients may have an inability to recognize that the beliefs associated with their obsessions are senseless and this may hinder the learning process that takes place during prolonged and repeated exposures to feared stimuli.

Because of the non-adherence issue with poor insight, cognitive therapy may be more useful initially to challenge the thoughts before using ERP.

Medication should also be started to see if by improving insight the person may then be more amenable to ERP.

PANDAS/PANS

The term Pediatric Autoimmune Neuropsychiatric Disorders Associated with Streptococcus infections (PANDAS) was coined to describe a subset of childhood obsessive compulsive disorders (OCD) and Tic Disorders triggered by group-A beta-hemolytic *Streptococcus pyogenes* infection. Pediatric Acute-onset Neuropsychiatric Syndrome (PANS) was later described to include a much broader category of behaviors and potential etiologies, including not only disorders potentially associated with a preceding infection, but also acute onset neuropsychiatric disorders without an apparent environmental precipitant or immune dysfunction. Because cases of PANS are defined clinically, the syndrome is expected to include a number of related disorders which have different etiologies but share a common clinical presentation—the lightning-like onset or recurrence of OCD accompanied by two or more co-occurring neuropsychiatric symptoms.

Despite advances in the knowledge of the pathogenesis of OCD, little is known about the causative mechanisms. Observations of patients with rheumatic fever who had Sydenham's chorea manifesting with classic OCD symptoms have suggested a possible etiological link between group A β-hemolytic *streptococcus* (GABHS) infection in a subset of OCD patients. GABHS has also been implicated in the development of Tourette's Syndrome and autism in children. Despite growing support for an association between GABHS and OCD, the causal relationship between GABHS infection and OCD, its pathophysiology, and its possible clinical implication remain highly controversial.

Clinical Presentation

Onset

Patients present with an abrupt and dramatic onset of OCD. The acuity of onset and initial severity of the OC symptoms are hallmarks of the diagnosis. The OCD symptoms must be sufficiently frequent and intense to meet DSM-5 criteria for OCD and must cause significant distress and interference in the child's activities at home, at school, and/or with peers.

Many parents describe the onset as the child waking up one day a different character. Many parents can pinpoint the exact date neuropsychiatric symptoms erupted and their child's personality changed from baseline.

A prior history of mild, non-impairing obsessions or compulsions does not, however, rule out the syndrome, as children may have had subclinical symptoms present for an extended period prior to the sudden onset of the full disorder.

Eating Disorder Symptoms

In addition to the initial OCD symptoms, there is also usually restricted food intake and abnormal eating behaviors. In some patients, body image distortions appear to drive the weight-loss inducing behaviors; while in the majority, the body image distortions appear only after the child had lost a significant amount of weight (10–15% of starting weight) as a result of food intake restrictions that were related to obsessional preoccupations with the texture of food and a fear of choking, vomiting, or contamination from ingesting specific foods. The sudden onset of eating restrictions or anorexic behaviors can occur even in the absence of more typical symptoms of OCD.

Other Symptoms

Other common co-morbid symptoms can include reactivity, rages, mood lability (including with manic aspect), night-time fears, cognitive defects, oppositional behavior, hyperactivity, and Attention Deficit Hyperactivity Disorder-like presentations.

Anxiety. The anxiety may manifest as either new-onset or a sudden exacerbation of separation anxiety, generalized anxiety, irrational fears or worries, or a specific phobia. Early in the course of illness, the child may appear "terror stricken," hyper-alert, and excessively vigilant. Over the course of several days to a few weeks, the apparent panic may subside to a state of generalized anxiety, with repeated requests for reassurance that the child did not do something wrong or that he or she is safe.

Emotional lability and depression. The child may experience sudden and unexpected changes in mood, often shifting from laughter to tears without obvious precipitants. The child may complain of restlessness and agitation, which is similarly un-precipitated and inexplicable.

Aggression, irritability, and oppositional behaviors. These symptoms are often the reason parents seek medical advice. The irritability and oppositional behaviors are present throughout the day and the aggression can occur without provocation. Most notable is the striking contrast between these new behaviors and the child's usual state.

Behavioral (developmental) regression. These symptoms include an abrupt increase in temper tantrums, loss of age-appropriate language (sometimes to the point of the child using "baby talk"), and other behaviors inappropriate to the child's chronological age and previous stage of development.

Sudden deterioration in school performance or learning abilities. A number of factors may contribute to the child's academic difficulties, including a shortened attention span, difficulties with concentration or memorization, specific losses of math skills or visuospatial skills, and other disturbances of cognition or executive functioning.

Sensory and motor abnormalities. The sensory abnormalities may include a sudden sensitivity to light, noises, smells, tastes or textures of foods, or items of clothing, or conversely, sensory-seeking behaviors, such as needing to touch or feel particular objects or textures. Visual hallucinations may also occur and might include frightening images and perceptions that objects are floating or that they are larger or smaller than actual size. Motor abnormalities occurring in PANS may include an abrupt deterioration of the child's handwriting (dysgraphia), clumsiness, motor hyperactivity, tics, and choreiform movements.

Somatic signs and symptoms. Sleep problems and disturbances of micturition (desire to urinate) and urination (the act itself) are among the most common physical manifestations of PANS.

Diagnosis

PANS is a clinical diagnosis, often marked by sudden onset and extreme symptom exacerbations. The diagnostic criteria for PANS include the following:

Criterion Description

I. An abrupt, dramatic onset of obsessive compulsive disorder and/or severely restricted food intake;
II. Concurrent occurrence of additional neuropsychiatric symptoms, with similarly severe and acute onset, from at least two of the following categories:
   1. Anxiety
   2. Emotional lability and/or depression

3. Irritability, aggression and/or severely oppositional behaviors
4. Behavioral (developmental) regression
5. Deterioration in school performance
6. Sensory or motor abnormalities
7. Somatic signs and symptoms, including sleep disturbances, enuresis, or urinary frequency

III. Symptoms are not readily explained better by a known neurologic or medical disorder, such as Sydenham chorea, systemic lupus erythematosus, or Tourette's Disorder.

Diagnostic Issues

When a child has primarily vocal and motor tics, the symptoms may appear to overlap with symptoms of Tourette's Syndrome; however, the children can be differentiated by observing symptom exacerbations over time.

In PANDAS/PANS children, a streptococcal infection may coincide with symptom exacerbation and once treated, initial exacerbations may generally remit. The rapid onset with significant remission is characteristic of PANDAS.

Researchers have described chronic PANDAS/PANS where the tics and/or OCD have a much more gradual improving course. These cases are difficult to separate from non-PANDAS/PANS tics or OCD. Some researchers have found other immunologic markers (anti-neuronal and anti-basal-ganglia antibodies) that help separate PANDAS and non-PANDAS children.

Diagnostic Tests

To make a diagnosis of PANS, clinicians must perform a diagnostic evaluation that is comprehensive enough to rule out other salient disorders, including toxic effects of drugs or medications, acute disseminated encephalomyelitis, and other neurologic disorders. The nature of the co-occurring symptoms will dictate the necessary assessments, which may include magnetic resonance imaging

(MRI) scan, lumbar puncture, electroencephalogram, and other diagnostic tests.

In addition, it may be useful to obtain a throat culture for streptococcal or serial antibody titers, or to perform other laboratory tests that might identify a treatable precipitant for the neuropsychiatric symptoms. At this time, there are no commercially available tests for diagnosing PANDAS/PANS.

A throat culture for Group A Beta-Hemolytic streptococcus (GABHS) at time of exacerbation onset is recommended to diagnose a pharyngeal streptococcal infection. If the culture is negative, blood tests may be able to test for streptococcal exotoxins. Common blood tests are Anti-Streptolycin O (ASO titer test) and the Anti D-NaseB titer test. While these tests can confirm a current or recent strep infection, they cannot exclude a prior infection or a diagnosis of PANDAS. These tests are affected by many factors and in one study over 46% of children did not have a rising ASO titer despite having colonized strep.

Titers have to be measured at two points (typically a week apart). ASO tends to rise 1–4 weeks post infection and anti-DNAseB tends to reach a peak at around 6–8 weeks. Therefore, ASO is typically measured at 4 and 5 weeks from the date of suspected infection and anti-DNAseB measured at 6 weeks and 8 weeks from the suspected event. The two data points are needed to look for a rise. Absolute values are not as important as the rise or fall of the titer. In the absence of having two titers, many labs use a measure known as the upper-limit-of-normal (ULN). This value is helpful if the measured value is significantly higher than the upper limit. If it is lower than the ULN, then typically two samples are needed to look at the slope/trend.

Low ASO titers do not rule out PANDAS/PANS. Although most strains of GABHS produce streptolycin-O, cholesterol can absorb this exotoxin. In one study, ASO did not rise in 46% of patients despite positive throat cultures and perfect timing for taking the ASO titer. So ASO can confirm a previous strep infection but cannot rule out strep or PANDAS/PANS. Similarly, a low anti-DNAseB titer does not rule out PANDAS/PANS.

For children affected by PANDAS/PANS, subsequent exacerbations may be triggered by recurrent GABHS or by other bacterial or viral infections (ear infections, sinusitis, pneumonia, meningitis, impetigo) further complicating diagnosis.

Differential Diagnosis

Other autoimmune illnesses that may cause sudden onset OCD include: Lyme disease, Thyroid disease, Celiac disease, Lupus, Sydenham Chorea, Kawasaki's disease, and acute Rheumatic Fever.

Some children have been found to have immunology deficits such as IgG subclass deficiencies. Children will need to be evaluated for this issue by an immunologist.

Treatment Strategies

Standard OCD Treatment

Standard therapies (SSRIs and cognitive behavioral therapy [CBT]) have some efficacy in the PANDAS/PANS subset of OCD, although well-controlled trials are lacking.

Studies of CBT have shown some efficacy with older PANDAS/PANS children, but the main benefit seems to be that parents learned techniques for managing OCD exacerbations.

Some research suggests that children with PANDAS/PANS may experience higher behavioral activation rates on SSRIs. Other reports, however, suggest that OCD in patients with PANDAS/PANS respond to serotonergic drugs. There are not controlled studies on the use of antipsychotic augmentation in children in the PANDAS/PANS subgroup.

Immunotherapies

If PANDAS and a streptococcal infection are suspected, the individual can be treated with antibiotics such as penicillin, amoxicillin, azithromycin, and augmentin (standard dosing). Penicillin, augmentin, and azithromycin appear to be more clinically effective in clearing GABHS than amoxicillin. In some cases, parents have reported a behavioral/symptomatic improvement within 24 hours. Most patients, however, appear to need 10–12 days of antibiotics for improvement. About 3 weeks after completing treatment for strep, a new culture can be drawn.

Prophylaxis with antibiotics may prevent exacerbations of future symptoms but raises concerns about antibiotic-resistance.

Other acute treatment options include immunomodulating therapy such as intravenous immunoglobulins (IVIG) and Plasmapheresis. Immunomodulating therapies do not appear to be effective for Tourette's Syndrome or other non-PANDAS OCD cases.

With IVIG, immunoglobulin antibodies, type G, are extracted from donated blood and transferred to the recipient through an intravenous line. IVIG is used in many auto-immune diseases but the exact nature of how it works is not known. IVIG is highly anti-inflammatory and may help T-regulatory cells become re-activated to help remove anti-host antibodies. In addition, some of the infused antibodies may help recognize infected cells or bacteria that were missed by the recipient's own antibodies. Expert neurological input is advised.

Plasmapheresis is a process of removing antibodies from the blood stream through filtration. Another donor's plasma is added on the return so that new antibodies are added (similar to IVIG). Plasmapheresis is used in severe auto-immune diseases because it can address acute antibody levels.

Some evidence suggests that both IVIG and plasmaphersis have better long-term outcomes when followed up with prophylactic antibiotic use.

Key References

- Nicholson TR, Ferdinando S, Krishnaiah RB, Anhoury S, Lennox BR, Mataix-Cols D, Cleare A, Veale DM, Drummond LM,

Fineberg NA, Church AJ, Giovannoni G, Heyman I. Prevalence of anti-basal ganglia antibodies in adult obsessive compulsive disorder: cross-sectional study. Br J Psychiatry. 2012 May;200(5):381–6.

- Shulman ST. Pediatric autoimmune neuropsychiatric disorders associated with streptococci (PANDAS): update. Curr Opin Pediatr. 2009 Feb;21(1):127–30.
- Snider LA, Swedo SE. PANDAS: current status and directions for research. Mol Psychiatry. 2004 Oct;9(10):900–7.

Appendix A

Suggested Further Reading

Note: This list comprises a number of books which clinicians and patients may find useful and interesting, however, it is not meant to be exhaustive.

Obsessive Compulsive Disorder

- Obsessive Compulsive Disorders: A Practical Guide: Management and Treatment (2001). Naomi Fineberg, Donatella Marazziti, and Dan Stein (ISBN-10: 1853179191; ISBN-13: 978-1853179198)
- Obsessive Compulsive Disorder (2007). Dan Stein and Naomi Fineberg (ISBN-10: 0199204608; ISBN-13: 978-0199204601)
- Exposure and Response (Ritual) Prevention for Obsessive Compulsive Disorder: Therapist Guide (Treatments That Work) (2012). Edna B. Foa, Elna Yadin, and Tracey K. Lichner (ISBN-10: 0195335287; ISBN-13: 978-0195335286)
- Getting Control: Overcoming Your Obsessions and Compulsions (2012). Lee Baer (ISBN-10: 9780452297852; ISBN-13: 978-0452297852)
- Brain Lock: Free Yourself from Obsessive Compulsive Behavior (1997). Jeffrey M. Schwartz and Beverly Beyette (ISBN-10: 0060987111; ISBN-13: 978-0060987114)

- The Boy Who Couldn't Stop Washing: The Experience and Treatment of Obsessive Compulsive Disorder (1991). Judith L. Rapoport (ISBN-10: 0451172027; ISBN-13: 978-0451172020)
- The Imp of the Mind: Exploring the Silent Epidemic of Obsessive Bad Thoughts (2006). Lee Baer (ISBN-10: 0452283078; ISBN-13: 978-0452283077)
- Obsessive Compulsive and Related Disorders in Adults: A Comprehensive Clinical Guide (1999). Lorrin Koran (ISBN-10: 0521559758)

Hoarding

- Compulsive Hoarding and Acquiring: Therapist Guide (Treatments That Work) (2006). Gail Steketee and Randy O. Frost (ISBN-10: 0195300254; ISBN-13: 978-0195300253)
- Overcoming Compulsive Hoarding: Why You Save and How You Can Stop (2004). Jerome Bubrick, Fugen Neziroglu, Jose Yaryura-Tobias, and Patricia B. Perkins (ISBN-10: 157224349X; ISBN-13: 978-1572243491)
- Buried in Treasures: Help for Compulsive Acquiring, Saving, and Hoarding (2007). David F. Tolin, Randy O. Frost, and Gail Steketee (ISBN-10: 0195300580; ISBN-13: 978-0195300581)

Body Dysmorphic Disorder

- The Broken Mirror: Understanding and Treating Body Dysmorphic Disorder (2005). Katherine A. Philips (ISBN-10: 0195167198, ISBN-13: 978-019516)
- Cognitive-Behavioral Therapy for Body Dysmorphic Disorder: A Treatment Manual (2012). Sabine Wilhelm, Katharine A. Phillips, and Gail Steketee (ISBN-10: 1462507905; ISBN-13: 978-1462507900)

- Overcoming Body Dysmorphic Disorder: A Cognitive Behavioral Approach to Reclaiming Your Life (2012). Fugen Neziroglu, Sony Khemlani-Patel, and Melanie T. Santos (ISBN-10: 1608821498; ISBN-13: 978-1608821495)
- Body Dysmorphic Disorder: A Treatment Manual (2010). David Veale and Fugen Neziroglu (ISBN-10: 047085121X; ISBN-13: 978-0470851210)

Hypochondriasis

- Hypochondriasis: Modern Perspectives on an Ancient Malady (2001). Vladan Starcevic and Don R. Lipsitt (ISBN-10: 0195126769; ISBN-13: 978-0195126761)
- Hypochondriasis and Health Anxiety, in the series Advances in Psychotherapy, Evidence Based Practice (2010). Jonathan Abramowitz and Autumn Braddock (ISBN-10: 0889373256; ISBN-13: 978-0889373259)

Trichotillomania and Excoriation (Skin Picking) Disorder

- Help for Hair Pullers: Understanding and Coping with Trichotillomania (2001). Nancy J. Keuthen, Dan J. Stein, and Gary A. Christenson (ISBN-10: 1572242329, ISBN-13: 978-1572242326)
- The Hair-pulling problem; A Complete Guide to Trichotillomania (2003). Fred Penzel (ISBN-10: 0195149424, ISBN-13: 978-0195149425)
- Trichotillomania, Skin Picking, and Other Body-focused Repetitive Behaviors (2011), Edited by Jon Grant, Dan Stein, Douglas Woods, and Nancy Keuthen (ISBN-10: 1585623989, ISBN-13: 978-1585623983)
- Trichotillomania: An ACT-enhanced Behavior Therapy Approach Therapist Guide (Treatments That Work) (2008). Douglas

W. Woods and Michael P. Twohig (ISBN-10: 0195336038; ISBN-13: 978-0195336030)
- The Hair Pulling "Habit" and You: How to Solve the Trichotillomania Puzzle, Revised Edition (2000). Ruth Goldfinger Golomb and Sherrie Mansfield Vavrichek (ISBN-10: 0967305020; ISBN-13: 978-0967305028)
- Treating Trichotillomania: Cognitive-Behavioral Therapy for Hairpulling and Related Problems (Series in Anxiety and Related Disorders) (2007). Martin E. Franklin and David F. Tolin (ISBN-10: 0387708820; ISBN-13: 978-0387708829)

Tic Disorders

- Treating Tourette Syndrome and Tic Disorders: A Guide for Practitioners (2007). Douglas W. Woods, John C. Piacentini, John T. Walkup, and Peter Hollenbeck (ISBN-10: 1593854803; ISBN-13: 978-1593854805)
- Managing Tourette Syndrome: A Behavioral Intervention for Children and Adults Therapist Guide (Treatments That Work) (2008). Douglas W. Woods, John Piacentini, Susanna Chang, and Thilo Deckersbach (ISBN-10: 0195341287; ISBN-13: 978-01953412)

Appendix B

Resources

Note: This list is not meant to be exhaustive but rather a reference to some key organizations and treatment centers in the United States and around the world.

Organizations

Name of Organization	*Website*	*Contact*
	USA	
International OCD Foundation	www.ocfoundation.org	**Mailing Address**: International OCD Foundation, Inc. P.O. Box 961029 Boston, MA 02196 **Phone**: 617-973-5801 **Email**: info@ocfoundation.org
Trichotillomania Learning Center	www.trich.org	**Mailing Address**: 207 McPherson Street, Suite H Santa Cruz, CA 95060 **Phone**: 831-457-1004 **Email**: info@trich.org
Tourette's Syndrome Association	www.tsa-usa.org	**Mailing Address**: 42-40 Bell Boulevard Bayside, NY 11361 **Phone**: 718-224-2999

National Alliance on Mental Illness	http://www.nami.org Locate a local NAMI contact in the US: http://www.nami.org/Template.cfm?Section=Your_Local_NAMI	**Mailing Address**: NAMI 3803 North Fairfax Drive, Suite 1000 Arlington, VA 22203 **Phone**: 800-950-6264
Obsessive Compulsive Disorder Clinic, Butler Hospital	http://www.butler.org/ocd-clinic/index.cfm	**Address**: 345 Blackstone Boulevard Providence, RI 02906 USA **Phone**: 401-455-6366
The Obsessive Compulsive Disorder Institute, McLean Hospital	http://www.mclean.harvard.edu/patient/adult/ocd.php	**Address**: 115 Mill Street Belmont, MA 02478 USA **Phone**: 800-333-0338
Addictive, Compulsive and Impulsive Disorders Research Program, University of Chicago	http://acid.uchicago.edu	**Address**: Department of Psychiatry 5841 S Maryland Avenue Chicago, IL 60637 USA **Phone**: 773-702-9066

(continued)

Name of Organization	*Website*	*Contact*
OCD and Related Disorders Program, Massachusetts General Hospital	https://mghocd.org/clinical-services/ocd	**Address**: MGH OCD and Related Disorders Program Richard B. Simches Research Ctr 185 Cambridge Street, Suite 2000 Boston, MA 02114 USA **Phone**: 617-726-6766
Center for OCD and Anxiety-Related Disorders Saint Louis Behavioral Medicine Institute	www.slbmi.com	**Address**: Center for OCD and Anxiety-Related Disorders Saint Louis Behavioral Medicine Institute 1129 Macklind Avenue St. Louis, MO 63105 **Phone**: 314-534-0200, Ext. 407 **Email**: mertenss@slbmi.com
SkinPicking.com	www.stoppicking.com	**Address**: 1832 Lexington Houston, TX 77098 USA **Email**: info@stoppicking.com

StopPulling.com	www.stoppulling.com	**Address**: 1832 Lexington Houston, TX 77098 USA **Email**: info@stoppulling.com
UK		
International College of Obsessive Compulsive Spectrum Disorders (ICOCS)	www.icocs.org	**Mailing Address**: ICOCS Devonshire House, Manor Way Borehamwood Hertfordshire, WD6 1QQ UK **Email**: office@icocs.org
Young People with OCD	http://www.ocdyouth.info	**Address**: Young People's OCD Clinic Michael Rutter Centre Maudsley Hospital Denmark Hill London SE5 8AZ **Email**: ocdyoutheditor@iop.kcl.ac.uk

(continued)

Name of Organization	*Website*	*Contact*
OCD UK	www.ocduk.org	**Address**: Virgin Care Limited Lynton House 7-12 Tavistock Square London, WC1H 9LT **Email**: support@ocduk.org **Phone**: 0845 120 3778
First Steps	www.firststeps-surrey.nhs.uk	**Address**: OCD-UK PO Box 8955 Nottingham, NG10 9AU **Email**: first.steps@nhs.net **Phone**: 0808 801 0325
OCD Action	www.ocdaction.org.uk	**Address**: OCD Action Suite 506-507 Davina House 137-149 Goswell Road London, EC1V 7ET **Email**: support@ocaction.org.uk **Phone**: 020 7253 5272 or 0845 390 6232

South Africa		
Mental Health Information Centre, Southern Africa	http://www.mentalhealthsa.co.za	**Address**: PO Box 19063 Tygerberg 7505 **Email**: mhic@sun.ac.za **Phone**: +27 21 938-9229
Canada		
The Ontario Obsessive Compulsive Disorder Network (OOCDN)	http://www.ocdontario.org/index.html	**Address**: 204 Sproule DriveBarrie Ontario L4N 0N4 **Email**: info@ocdontario.org **Phone**: 416-410-4772
Australia		
Anxiety Recovery Centre Victoria	www.arcvic.com.au/index.html	**Address**: P.O Box 367 Canterbury Vic 3126 **Phone**: 03 9830 0533 or 1300 ANXIETY
Anxiety & Stress Management Service of Australia	www.anxietyhelp.com.au	**Address**: P.O Box 94 Indooroopilly QLD, Australia 4068 **Email**: contact@anxietyhelp.com.au

Appendix C

Scales

Body Dysmorphic Disorder Modification of the Y-BOCS (BDD-YBOCS) (Adult version)

For each item circle the number of the response which best characterizes the patient during the **past week.**

1. Time Occupied by Thoughts about Body Defect

How much of your time is occupied by THOUGHTS about a defect or flaw in your appearance [list body parts of concern]?

0 = None
1 = Mild (less than 1 hr/day)
2 = Moderate (1–3 hr/day)
3 = Severe (greater than 3 and up to 8 hr/day)
4 = Extreme (greater than 8 hr/day)

2. Interference Due to Thoughts About Body Defect

How much do your THOUGHTS about your body defect(s) interfere with your social or work (role) functioning? (Is there anything you aren't doing or can't do because of them?)

Examples include:

Y/N Spending time with friends
Y/N Dating
Y/N Attending social functions
Y/N Doing things w/family in and outside of home
Y/N Going to school/work each day
Y/N Being on time for or missing school/work
Y/N Focusing at school/work
Y/N Productivity at school/work
Y/N Doing homework or maintaining grades
Y/N Daily activities

0 = None
1 = Mild, slight interference with social, occupational, or role activities, but overall performance not impaired
2 = Moderate, definite interference with social, occupational, or role performance, but still manageable
3 = Severe, causes substantial impairment in social, occupational, or role performance
4 = Extreme, incapacitating

3. Distress Associated with thoughts about Body Defect

How much distress do your THOUGHTS about your body defect(s) cause you?

Rate "disturbing" feelings or anxiety that seem to be triggered by these thoughts, not general anxiety or anxiety associated with other symptoms.

0 = None
1 = Mild, not too disturbing
2 = Moderate, disturbing
3 = Severe, very disturbing
4 = Extreme, disabling distress

4. Resistance Against thoughts of Body Defect

How much of an effort do you make to resist these THOUGHTS?

How often do you try to disregard them or turn your attention away from these thoughts as they enter your mind?

Only rate effort made to resist, NOT success or failure in actually controlling the thoughts. How much patient resists the thoughts may or may not correlate with ability to control them.

0 = Makes an effort to always resist, or symptoms so minimal doesn't need to actively resist
1 = Tries to resist most of time
2 = Makes some effort to resist
3 = Yields to all such thoughts without attempting to control them but yields with some reluctance
4 = Completely and willingly yields to all such thoughts

5. Degree of control over thoughts about Body Defect

How much control do you have over your THOUGHTS about your body defect(s)?

How successful are you in stopping or diverting these thoughts?

0 = Complete control, or no need for control because thoughts are so minimal
1 = Much control, usually able to stop or divert these thoughts with some effort and concentration
2 = Moderate control, sometimes able to stop or divert these thoughts
3 = Little control, rarely successful in stopping thoughts, can only divert attention with difficulty
4 = No control, experienced as completely involuntary, rarely able to even momentarily divert attention

6. Time Spent in Activities Related to Body Defect

The next several questions are about the activities/behaviors you do in relation to your body defects.

How much time do you spend in ACTIVITIES related to your concern over your appearance?

0 = None
1 = Mild (spends less than 1 hr/day)
2 = Moderate (1-3 hrs/day)
3 = Severe (spends more than 3 and up to 8 hours/day)
4 = Extreme (spends more than 8 hrs/day)

Go through list of activities with patient (ask questions 6-10 about all that apply)

___Checking mirrors/other surfaces
___Grooming activities
___Applying makeup
___Excessive exercise (time beyond 1 hr a day)
___Selecting/changing clothing or other cover-up (rate time spent selecting/changing clothes, not time wearing them)
___Scrutinizing others' appearance (comparing)
___Questioning others about or discussing your appearance
___Picking at skin
___Touching the body areas
___Other ______________________

7. Interference Due to Activities Related to Body Defect

How much do these ACTIVITIES interfere with your social or work (role) functioning? (Is there anything you don't do because of them?)

0 = None
1 = Mild, slight interference with social, occupational, or role activities, but overall performance not impaired
2 = Moderate, definite interference with social, occupational, or role performance, but still manageable
3 = Severe, causes substantial impairment in social, occupational, or role performance
4 = Extreme, incapacitating

8. Distress Associated with Activities Related to Body Defect

How would you feel if you were prevented from performing these ACTIVITIES?

How anxious would you become?

Rate degree of distress/frustration patient would experience if performance of the activities were suddenly interrupted.

0 = None
1 = Mild, only slightly anxious if behavior prevented
2 = Moderate, reports that anxiety would mount but remain manageable if behavior is prevented
3 = Severe, prominent and very disturbing increase in anxiety if behavior is interrupted
4 = Extreme, incapacitating anxiety from any intervention aimed at modifying activity

9. Resistance against Compulsions

How much of an effort do you make to resist these ACTIVITIES?

Only rate effort made to resist, NOT success or failure in actually controlling the activities.

How much the patient resists these behaviors may or may not correlate with his/her ability to control them.

0 = Makes an effort to always resist, or symptoms so minimal doesn't need to actively resist
1 = Tries to resist most of the time
2 = Makes some effort to resist
3 = Yields to almost all of these behaviors without attempting to control them, but does so with some reluctance
4 = Completely and willingly yields to all behaviors related to body defect

10. Degree of Control over Compulsive behavior

How strong is the drive to perform these behaviors? How much control do you have over them?

0 = Complete control, or control is unnecessary because symptoms are mild
1 = Much control, experiences pressure to perform the behavior, but usually able to exercise voluntary control over it
2 = Moderate control, strong pressure to perform behavior, can control it only with difficulty
3 = Little control, very strong drive to perform behavior, must be carried to completion, can delay only with difficulty
4 = No control, drive to perform behavior experienced as completely involuntary and overpowering, rarely able to even momentarily delay activity

11. Insight

Is it possible that your defect might be less noticeable or less unattractive than you think it is?

How convinced are you that [fill in body part] is as unattractive as you think it is?

Can anyone convince you that it doesn't look so bad?

0 = Excellent insight, fully rational
1 = Good insight. Readily acknowledges absurdity of thoughts (but doesn't seem completely convinced that there isn't something besides anxiety to be concerned about)
2 = Fair insight. Reluctantly admits that thoughts seem unreasonable but wavers
3 = Poor insight. Maintains that thoughts are not unreasonable
4 = Lacks insight, delusional. Definitely convinced that concerns are reasonable, unresponsive to contrary evidence

12. Avoidance

Have you been avoiding doing anything, going any place, or being with anyone because of your thoughts or behaviors related to your body defects?

If YES, then ask: What do you avoid?

Rate degree to which patient deliberately tries to avoid things such as social interactions or work-related activities. Do not include avoidance of mirrors or avoidance of compulsive behaviors.

0 = No deliberate avoidance
1 = Mild, minimal avoidance
2 = Moderate, some avoidance clearly present
3 = Severe, much avoidance; avoidance prominent
4 = Extreme, very extensive avoidance; patient avoids almost all activities

Brackets [ ] indicate material that should be read, filling in the body parts of concern.
Parentheses () in the probes indicate optional material that may be read.
Italicized items are instructions and reminders to the interviewer.

 Source: Phillips KA, Hollander E, Rasmussen SA, Aronowitz BR, DeCaria C, et al. A severity rating scale for Body Dysmorphic Disorder: development, reliability, and validity of a modified version of the Yale-Brown Obsessive Compulsive Scale. Psychopharmacol Bull. 1997;33:17–22.

Hoarding Rating Scale

Please use the following scale when answering items below:

0 = no problem
2 = mild problem, occasionally (less than weekly) acquires items not needed, or acquires a few unneeded items
4 = moderate, regularly (once or twice weekly) acquires items not needed, or acquires some unneeded items

6 = severe, frequently (several times per week) acquires items not needed, or acquires many unneeded items
8 = extreme, very often (daily) acquires items not needed, or acquires large numbers of unneeded items

1. Because of the clutter or number of possessions, how difficult is it for you to use the rooms in your home?

0	1	2	3	4	5	6	7	8
Not at all Difficult		Mild		Moderate		Severe		Extremely Difficult

2. To what extent do you have difficulty discarding (or recycling, selling, giving away) ordinary things that other people would get rid of?

0	1	2	3	4	5	6	7	8
No difficulty		Mild		Moderate		Severe		Extreme Difficulty

3. To what extent do you currently have a problem with collecting free things or buying more things than you need or can use or can afford?

0	1	2	3	4	5	6	7	8
None		Mild		Moderate		Severe		Extreme

4. To what extent do you experience emotional distress because of clutter, difficulty discarding, or problems with buying or acquiring things?

0	1	2	3	4	5	6	7	8
None/ Not at all		Mild	Moderate		Severe		Extreme	

5. To what extent do you experience impairment in your life (daily routine, job/school, social activities, family activities, financial difficulties) because of clutter, difficulty discarding, or problems with buying or acquiring things?

0	1	2	3	4	5	6	7	8
None/ Not at all		Mild	Moderate		Severe		Extreme	

Interpretation of HRS Total Scores (Tolin et al., 2010)
Mean for nonclinical samples: HRS Total = 3.34; standard deviation = 4.97.

Mean for people with hoarding problems: HRS Total = 24.22; standard deviation = 5.67.

Analysis of sensitivity and specificity suggest an HRS Total clinical cutoff score of 14.

Criteria for Clinically Significant Hoarding (Tolin et al., 2008)

A score of 4 or greater on questions 1 and 2, and a score of 4 or greater on either question 4 or question 5.

Hypochondriasis Yale-Brown Obsessive Compulsive Scale Modified (H-YBOCS-M)

Rating Interval—the Last 2 Weeks

Illness Thoughts or Worries (items 1–6)

"I am now going to ask several questions about your concerns that you have or might have a serious illness or disease." (Make specific reference to the patient's target illness worries and thoughts.)

1. Time occupied by worries related to illness or disease

Q: When you have a day with worries that you have or might have a serious disease or worry about a symptom suggestive of serious disease, how much time do these worries last, if you add up all the illness worries of the day? What's the average total worry duration if you look at each of the days afflicted by worry?

0 = None
1 = Mild amount of time: less than 1 hr/day
2 = Moderate amount of time: 1 to 3 hr/day
3 = Severe amount of time: greater than 3 and up to 8 hr/day
4 = Extreme amount of time: greater than 8 hr/day or nearly constant

2. Frequency of worries related to illness or disease

Q: How often have you had thoughts that you have or might have an illness or serious disease or worried about a symptom suggestive to you of a serious disease (in last 2 weeks)?

0 = None
1 = Seldom: less than 1 × week
2 = Sometimes: 1–3 × week
3 = Often: 4–6 × week
4 = Very often: Daily

3. Interference due to thoughts related to illness or disease

Q: How much do your worries about illness or serious disease interfere with your social or work (or role) functioning? Is there anything that you don't do because your mind is so preoccupied with thoughts about illness? [If currently not working, determine how much performance would be affected if patient were employed.]

0 = None
1 = Mild, slight interference with social or occupational activities, but overall performance not impaired
2 = Moderate, definite interference with social or occupational performance, but still manageable
3 = Severe, causes substantial impairment in social or occupational performance
4 = Extreme, incapacitating

4. Distress associated with thoughts related to illness or disease

Q: How much distress do your thoughts about illness or serious disease cause you? [In most cases, distress is equated with anxiety. Only rate anxiety that seems triggered by illness/disease thoughts, not generalized anxiety or anxiety associated with other conditions.]

0 = None
1 = Mild, not too disturbing
2 = Moderate, disturbing, but still manageable
3 = Severe, very disturbing
4 = Extreme, near constant and disabling distress

5. Resistance against thoughts related to illness or disease

Q: When you have a symptom suggestive of a serious disease or the thought of having an illness, how much of an effort do you make to resist the thoughts about illness or serious disease—to put them out of your mind—to distract yourself? [Only rate effort made to resist, not success or failure in putting them out of mind.]

0 = Makes an effort to always resist, or symptoms so minimal doesn't need to actively resist
1 = Tries to resist most of the time
2 = Makes some effort to resist the thoughts
3 = Yields to almost all thoughts without attempting to distract oneself, but does so with some reluctance
4 = Completely and willingly focuses on the thoughts of possibly having a serious disease

6. Degree of control over thoughts related to illness or disease

Q: When you think you have or might have a serious illness or experience a symptom that makes you worry you might have a serious illness, how much control do you have over your illness thoughts? How successful are you in stopping or diverting your concerns about illness? Can you dismiss them?

0 = Complete control
1 = Much control, usually able to stop or divert illness thoughts with some effort and concentration
2 = Moderate control, sometimes able to stop or divert illness thoughts

3 = Little control, rarely successful in stopping or dismissing thoughts about illness, can only divert attention with difficulty
4 = No control, experienced as completely involuntary, rarely able to even momentarily alter worries about illness and symptoms

Total for illness-related thoughts:__________________________

Illness-Related behaviors

"The next several questions are about behaviors that you perform in response to your concerns that you have or might have a serious illness or disease." (Reminder: Make specific reference to the patient's target illness behaviors. Make a clear distinction between active purposeful behaviors and avoidance. Do not include avoidance.)

7. Time occupied by behaviors related to illness concerns

Q: When you have a day when illness concerns arise, on average if you put all of the illness-related behaviors together for that particular day, how much time would it take? [These must be observable behaviors. For this scale, silent mental reviewing does not count as a compulsive behavior.]
0 = None
1 = Mild amount of time: less than 1 hr/day
2 = Moderate amount of time: 1 to 3 hr/day
3 = Severe amount of time: greater than 3 and up to 8 hr/day
4 = Extreme amount of time: greater than 8 hr/day or nearly constant

8. Frequency of behaviors related to your illness concerns

Q: How often have you had behaviors related to your concerns that you have or might have a serious illness?
0 = None
1 = Seldom: less than 1 × week
2 = Sometimes: 1–3 × week
3 = Often: 4–6 × week
4 = Very often: Daily

9. Interference due to behaviors in response to illness concerns

Q: How much does your behavior in response to illness concern interfere with your social or work (or role) functioning? [If currently not working, determine how much performance would be affected if patient were employed.]

0 = None

1 = Mild, slight interference with social or occupational activities, but overall performance not impaired

2 = Moderate, definite interference with social or occupational performance, but still manageable

3 = Severe, causes substantial impairment in social or occupational performance

4 = Extreme, incapacitating

10. Distress associated with behaviors in response to illness concerns

Q: How would you feel if you were prevented from performing an illness-related behavior? How would you feel if you were prevented from checking or from seeking reassurance? How anxious would you become?

0 = None

1 = Mild, only slightly anxious if behaviors were prevented

2 = Moderate, anxiety would mount but remain manageable

3 = Severe and very disturbing increase in anxiety if behaviors were prevented or interrupted

4 = Extreme, incapacitating anxiety from any intervention aimed at preventing behaviors or reassurance seeking

11. Resistance against behaviors related to illness concerns

Q: How much of an effort do you make to resist the illness-related behaviors? [Only rate effort made to resist, not success or failure in actually controlling the behaviors]?

0 = Makes an effort to always resist, or symptoms so minimal doesn't need to actively resist

1 = Tries to resist most of the time

2 = Makes some effort to resist

3 = Yields to almost all behaviors without attempting to control them, but does so with some reluctance

4 = Completely and willingly yields to all behaviors aimed at reducing illness concerns

12. Degree of control over behaviors related to illness concerns

Q: How strong is the drive to perform the illness-related behavior? How much control do you have over your illness-related behaviors? How successful are you in stopping or diverting your behaviors?

0 = Complete control

1 = Much control, experiences pressure to perform behavior but usually able to exercise voluntary control over it

2 = Moderate control, strong pressure to perform behavior, can control it only with difficulty

3 = Little control, very strong drive to perform the behavior. Must be carried to completion, but sometimes the behavior can be delayed

4 = No control, experienced as completely involuntary, rarely able to even momentarily divert the behavior

Total for illness-related behaviors: ______________________________

Illness-Related unhealthy avoidance

The remaining questions are about avoidance of situations following from fears or conviction of illness. Please note that *this refers to unhealthy avoidance.* In other words, this is avoidance stemming from fear of exposure to situations that a healthy person would not avoid. If avoidance is a healthy behavior for the patient, then it should not be considered "unhealthy avoidance" and should not be rated here. If a feared situation is not normally encountered, please ask the patient to rate the following items as if the opportunity for exposure to that situation was present on a daily basis. (Make specific references to the patient's avoidance behaviors.)

13. Extent of avoidance related to illness concerns

Q: How many different situations would you currently avoid (if placed in that situation) that are related to your concerns that you might have a serious illness or disease? [See the checklist for typical avoidance. Situations are overall themes, e.g., avoidance of physical exertion would be one theme that includes not taking the stairs, avoiding exercise or running after a bus, etc.]

0 = None

1 = Minimal: no more than one situation

2 = Moderate: two or three situations

3 = Severe: many situations
4 = Extreme: every situation that had any reminder of illness, death, or disease

14. Frequency of avoidance related to illness concerns
Q: How many days during the week would you now seek to avoid illness-related situations or reminders? [If the situation is not normally encountered, ask if avoidance would occur if encountered (hypothetically)?]
0 = None
1 = Seldom: less than 1 × week
2 = Sometimes: 1–3 × week
3 = Often: 4–6 × week
4 = Very often: daily (as often as possible)

15. Interference due to avoidance
Q: How much do your avoidance behaviors related to concerns about serious illness or disease interfere with your social or work (or role) functioning or with obtaining appropriate medical monitoring? In other words, by avoiding or not doing things, are you limiting your social or work life or potentially harming your own health? [Rate the avoidance that causes the most interference.]
0 = None
1 = Mild, slight interference with social or occupational activities or medical monitoring, but overall performance or health evaluations not impaired
2 = Moderate, definite interference with social or occupational performance or medical monitoring, but still manageable and does get medical check-ups every few years or if absolutely needed
3 = Severe, causes substantial impairment in social or occupational performance or medical monitoring is impaired (because person avoids getting tests that are recommended or needed)
4 = Extreme, incapacitating interference with social or work functioning or medical care (i.e., would not go for medical care even if one were quite ill or if there was a strong suspicion one were medically ill...or would not go to a hospital if that were part of one's job)

16. Distress associated with exposure to the avoided situation

Q: How would you feel if you were prevented from avoiding these situations or if you were asked not to avoid? How anxious would you become? [Rate degree of distress patient would experience if exposed to the avoided situation without being able to get reassurance. Rate the situation most feared or associated with the greatest distress.]

0 = None

1 = Mild only slightly anxious if exposed to the avoided situation

2 = Moderate, reports that anxiety would mount but remain manageable if exposed to the avoided situation or that anxiety increases but remains manageable

3 = Severe, prominent, and very disturbing increase in anxiety if exposed to the avoided situation

4 = Extreme, incapacitating anxiety if exposed to the avoided situation

17. Resistance against avoidance

Q: How much of an effort do you make to resist the avoidance (i.e., allow exposure of oneself to the illness-related situations)? [Only rate effort made to resist the avoidance, not success or failure in actually controlling the avoidance.]

0 = Makes an effort to *always* resist, or symptoms so minimal doesn't need to actively resist

1 = Tries to resist the avoidance of illness-related situations *most of the time*

2 = *Makes some effort* to resist the avoidance of illness-related situations

3 = *Yields to almost all avoidance* without attempting to control it, but does so with some reluctance (i.e., would avoid exposure to feared situation but with some reluctance)

4 = Completely and willingly yields to all illness-related avoidance

18. Degree of control over illness-related unhealthy avoidance

Q: How strong is the drive to avoid exposure to the feared situation? How much control do you have over the avoidance?

0 = Complete control

1 = Much control, experiences pressure, but usually able to allow exposure.

2 = Moderate control, strong pressure to avoid exposure, can prevent it only with difficulty
3 = Little control, very strong drive to avoid exposure, can only allow it with extreme difficulty
4 = No control, the need to avoid exposure is completely overpowering

Total for illness-related avoidance: ____________________

19. Insight into illness-related obsessive thoughts

Q: How often do you think your concerns or behaviors are unreasonable? What part of the time do you realize your illness worries are unreasonable?

0 = Excellent insight, evaluates illness-related obsessive thoughts always as unreasonable
1 = Good insight, evaluates illness-related obsessive thoughts as unreasonable most of the time (≥ 75% of the time)
2 = Fair insight, evaluates illness-related obsessive thoughts as unreasonable much of the time (≥50%, but <75% of the time)
3 = Poor insight, evaluates illness-related obsessive thoughts as unreasonable only some of the time (≥25%, but <50% of the time)
4 = Rare insight, rarely evaluates the illness-related obsessive thoughts as unreasonable (<25% of the time)

Total for illness thoughts/concerns (items 1–6): ____________
Total for illness-related behaviors (items 7–12): ____________
Total for items 1–12: ____________
Total for illness-related avoidance (items 13–18): ____________
Grand total (items 1–18): ____________

 Source: Skritskaya NA, Carson-Wong AR, Moeller JR, Shen S, Barsky AJ, Fallon BA. A clinician-administered severity rating scale for illness anxiety: development, reliability, and validity of the H-YBOCS-M. Depress Anxiety. 2012 Jul;29(7):652–64.

The Massachusetts General Hospital (MGH) Hairpulling Scale

Instructions: For each question, pick the one statement in that group which best describes your behaviors and/or feelings over the past week. If you have been having ups and downs, try to estimate an average for the past week. Be sure to read all the statements in each group before making your choice.

For the next three questions, rate only the urges to pull your hair.

1. **Frequency of urges.** On an average day, how often did you feel the urge to pull your hair?
   0 This week I felt no urges to pull my hair.
   1 This week I felt an **occasional** urge to pull my hair.
   2 This week I felt an urge to pull my hair **often.**
   3 This week I felt an urge to pull my hair **very often.**
   4 This week I felt **near constant** urges to pull my hair.

2. **Intensity of urges.** On an average day, how intense or "strong" were the urges to pull your hair?
   0 This week I did not feel any urges to pull my hair.
   1 This week I felt **mild** urges to pull my hair.
   2 This week I felt **moderate** urges to pull my hair.
   3 This week I felt **severe** urges to pull my hair.
   4 This week I felt **extreme** urges to pull my hair.

3. **Ability to control the urges.** On an average day, how much control do you have over the urges to pull your hair?
   0 This week I could **always** control the urges, or I did not feel any urges to pull my hair.
   1 This week I was always able to distract myself from the urges to pull my hair **most of the time.**
   2 This week I was able to distract myself from the urges to pull my hair **some of the time.**
   3 This week I was able to distract myself from the urges to pull my hair **rarely.**

4 This week I was **never** able to distract myself from the urges to pull my hair.

For the next three questions, rate only the actual hairpulling.

4. **Frequency of hairpulling.** On an average day, how often did you actually pull your hair?
   0 This week I did not pull my hair.
   1 This week I pulled my hair **occasionally.**
   2 This week I pulled my hair **often.**
   3 This week I pulled my hair **very often.**
   4 This week I pulled my hair so often it felt like I was **always** doing it.

5. **Attempts to resist hairpulling.** On an average day, how often did you make an attempt to stop yourself from actually pulling your hair?
   0 This week I felt no urges to pull my hair.
   1 This week I tried to resist the urge to pull my hair **almost all of the time.**
   2 This week I tried to resist the urge to pull my hair **some of the time.**
   3 This week I tried to resist the urge to pull my hair **rarely.**
   4 This week I **never** tried to resist the urge to pull my hair.

6. **Control over hairpulling.** On an average day, how often were you successful at actually stopping yourself from pulling your hair?
   0 This week I did not pull my hair.
   1 This week I was able to resist pulling my hair **almost all of the time.**
   2 This week I was able to resist pulling my hair **most of the time.**
   3 This week I was able to resist pulling my hair **some of the time.**
   4 This week I was **rarely** able to resist pulling my hair.

For the last question, rate the consequences of your hairpulling.

7. **Associated distress.** Hairpulling can make some people feel moody, "on edge," or sad. During the past week, how uncomfortable did your hairpulling make you feel?
   0 This week I did not feel uncomfortable about my hairpulling.
   1 This week I felt **vaguely uncomfortable** about my hairpulling.
   2 This week I felt **noticeably uncomfortable** about my hairpulling.
   3 This week I felt **significantly uncomfortable** about my hairpulling.
   4 This week I felt **intensely uncomfortable** about my hairpulling.

The Yale Global Tic Severity Scale

A. Instructions

This clinical rating scale is designed to rate the overall severity of tic symptoms across a range of dimensions (number, frequency, intensity, complexity, and interference). Use of the YGTSSS requires the rater to have clinical experience with Tourette's Syndrome patients. The final rating is based on all available information and reflects the clinician's overall impression for each of the items to be rated.

The style of the interview is semistructured. The interviewer should first complete the Tic Inventory (a list of motor and phonic tics present during the past week, as reported by the parent/patient, and observed during the evaluation). It is then best to proceed with questions based on each of the individual items, using the content of the anchor points as a guide.

B. Tic Inventory

1. *Description of Motor Tics:* (Check motor tics present during past week)

	a. *Simple Motor Tics:* (Rapid, Darting, "Meaningless"):
_____	Eye blinking
_____	Eye movements
_____	Nose movements
_____	Mouth movements
_____	Facial grimace
_____	Head jerks/movements
_____	Shoulder shrugs
_____	Arm movements
_____	Hand movements
_____	Abdominal tensing
_____	Leg or foot or toe movements
_____	Other ________________________________
_____	________________________________
_____	________________________________
	b. *Complex Motor Tics:* (Slower, "Purposeful"):
_____	Eye gestures or movements
_____	Mouth movements
_____	Facial movements or expressions
_____	Head gestures or movements

_____	Shoulder gestures
_____	Arm or hand gestures
_____	Writing tics
_____	Dystonic postures
_____	Bending or gyrating
_____	Rotating
_____	Leg or foot or toe movements
_____	Tic-related compulsive behaviors (touching, tapping, grooming, evening-up)
_____	Copropraxia
_____	Self-abusive behavior (describe)_____________________
_____	____
_____	Paroxysms of tics (displays), duration _________seconds
_____	Disinhibited behavior (describe)* ____________________
_____	____
_____	Other ____
_____	____
_____	Describe any orchestrated patterns or sequences of motor tic behaviors ____
_____	____

**Do not include this item in rating the ordinal scales.*

2. *Description of Phonic Tic Symptoms:* (Check phonic tics present over the past week)

_____	a. *Simple Phonic Symptoms:* (Fast, "Meaningless" Sounds):
	Sounds, noises: (circle: coughing, throat clearing, sniffing, grunting, whistling, animal or bird noises) Other (list) ______________________
_____	______________________________________
	b. *Complex Phonic Symptoms:* (Language: Words, Phrases, Statements):
_____	Syllables: (list) ______________________
_____	Words: (list) ______________________
_____	Coprolalia: (list) ______________________
_____	Echolalia ______________________
_____	Palalalia ______________________
_____	Blocking ______________________
_____	Speech atypicalities: (describe) ______________________
_____	______________________________________
_____	Disinhibited speech: (describe)* ______________________
_____	______________________________________
_____	Describe any orchestrated patterns or sequences of phonic tic behaviors ____
_____	______________________________________

C. *Ordinal Scales* (Rate motor and phonic tics separately unless otherwise indicated)

a. *Number:* Motor Score: [ ] Phonic Score: [ ]

Score	*Description (Anchor Point)*
0	None
1	Single tic
2	Multiple discrete tics (2–5)
3	Multiple discrete tics (>5)
4	Multiple discrete tics plus at least one orchestrated pattern of multiple simultaneous or sequential tics where it is difficult to distinguish discrete tics.
5	Multiple discrete tics plus several (>2) orchestrated patterns of multiple simultaneous or sequential tics where it is difficult to distinguish discrete tics.

b. *Frequency:* Motor Score: [ ] Phonic Score: [ ]

Score	*Description (Anchor Point)*
0	*None.* No evidence of specific tic behaviors.
1	*Rarely.* Specific tic behaviors have been present during previous week. These behaviors occur infrequently, often not on a daily basis. If bouts of tics occur, they are brief and uncommon.
2	*Occasionally.* Specific tic behaviors are usually present on a daily basis, but there are long tic-free intervals during the day. Bouts of tics may occur on occasion and are not sustained for more than a few minutes at a time.
3	*Frequently.* Specific tic behaviors are present on a daily basis. Tic-free intervals as long as 3 hours are not uncommon. Bouts of tics occur regularly but may be limited to a single setting.

4	*Almost Always.* Specific tic behaviors are present virtually every waking hour of every day, and periods of sustained tic behaviors occur regularly. Bouts of tics are common and are not limited to a single setting.
5	*Always.* Specific tic behaviors are present virtually all the time. Tic-free intervals are difficult to identify and do not last more than 5 to 10 minutes at most.

c. *Intensity:* Motor Score: [ ] Phonic Score: [ ]

Score	*Description (Anchor Point)*
0	*Absent*
1	*Minimal intensity,* tics not visible or audible (based solely on patient's private experience) or tics are less forceful than comparable voluntary actions and are typically not noticed because of their intensity.
2	*Mild intensity,* tics are not more forceful than comparable voluntary actions or utterances and are typically not noticed because of their intensity.
3	*Moderate intensity,* tics are more forceful than comparable voluntary actions but are not outside the range of normal expression for comparable voluntary actions or utterances. They may call attention to the individual because of their forceful character.
4	*Marked intensity,* tics are more forceful than comparable voluntary actions or utterances and typically have an "exaggerated" character. Such tics frequently call attention to the individual because of their forceful and exaggerated character.
5	*Severe intensity,* tics are extremely forceful and exaggerated in expression. These tics call attention to the individual and may result in risk of physical injury (accidental, provoked, or self-inflicted) because of their forceful expression.

d. *Complexity:* Motor Score: [ ] Phonic Score: [ ]

Score	*Description (Anchor Point)*
0	*None,* if present, all tics are clearly "simple" (sudden, brief, purposeless) in character.
1	*Borderline,* some tics are not clearly "simple" in character.
2	*Mild,* some tics are clearly "complex" (purposive in appearance) and mimic brief "automatic" behaviors, such as grooming, syllables, or brief meaningful utterances such as "ah huh," "hi," that could be readily camouflaged.
3	*Moderate,* some tics are more "complex" (more purposive and sustained in appearance) and may occur in orchestrated bouts that would be difficult to camouflage but could be rationalized or "explained" as normal behavior or speech (picking, tapping, saying "you bet" or "honey," brief echolalia).
4	*Marked,* some tics are very "complex" in character and tend to occur in sustained orchestrated bouts that would be difficult to camouflage and could not be easily rationalized as normal behavior or speech because of their duration and/or their unusual, inappropriate, bizarre, or obscene character (a lengthy facial contortion, touching genitals, echolalia, speech atypicalities, longer bouts of saying "what do you mean" repeatedly, or saying "fu" or "sh").
5	*Severe,* some tics involve lengthy bouts of orchestrated behavior or speech that would be impossible to camouflage or successfully rationalize as normal because of their duration and/or extremely unusual, inappropriate, bizarre, or obscene character (lengthy displays or utterances often involving copropraxia, self-abusive behavior, or coprolalia).

e. *Interference:* Motor Score: [ ] Phonic Score: [ ]

Score	*Description (Anchor Point)*
0	*None*
1	*Minimal,* when tics are present, they do not interrupt the flow of behavior or speech.
2	*Mild,* when tics are present, they occasionally interrupt the flow of behavior or speech.
3	*Moderate,* when tics are present, they frequently interrupt the flow of behavior or speech.
4	*Marked,* when tics are present, they frequently interrupt the flow of behavior or speech, and they occasionally disrupt intended action or communication.
5	*Severe,* when tics are present, they frequently disrupt intended action or communication.

f. *Impairment:* Overall Impairment: [ ] (Rate Overall Impairment for Motor and Phonic Tics)

Score	*Description (Anchor Point)*
0	*None*
10	*Minimal,* tics associated with subtle difficulties in self-esteem, family life, social acceptance, or school or job functioning (infrequent upset or concern about tics vis à vis the future; periodic, slight increase in family tensions because of tics; friends or acquaintances may occasionally notice or comment about tics in an upsetting way).
20	*Mild,* tics associated with minor difficulties in self-esteem, family life, social acceptance, or school or job functioning.

30	*Moderate,* tics associated with some clear problems in self-esteem, family life, social acceptance, or school or job functioning (episodes of dysphoria, periodic distress and upheaval in the family, frequent teasing by peers or episodic social avoidance, periodic interference in school or job performance because of tics).
40	*Marked,* tics associated with major difficulties in self-esteem, family life, social acceptance, or school or job functioning.
50	*Severe,* tics associated with extreme difficulties in self-esteem, family life, social acceptance, or school or job functioning (sever depression with suicidal ideation, disruption of the family [separation/divorce, residential placement], disruption of social ties—severely restricted life because of social stigma and social avoidance, removal from school or loss of job).

D. *Score Sheet*

Motor Tics:

Number	[ ]
Frequency	[ ]
Intensity	[ ]
Complexity	[ ]
Interference	[ ]
Total Motor Tic Score	[ ]

Phonic Tics:

Number	[ ]
Frequency	[ ]
Intensity	[ ]
Complexity	[ ]

Interference	[ ]
Total Phonic Tic Score	[ ]
Overall Impairment Rating	[ ]

Global Severity Score (Motor + Phonic + Impairment) [ ]

Reprinted with permission from Elsevier. Source: Leckman JF, Riddle MA, Hardin MT, Ort SI, Swartz KL, Stevenson J, Cohen DJ. The Yale Global Tic Severity Scale: initial testing of a clinician-rated scale of tic severity. J Am Acad Child Adolesc Psychiatry. 1989 Jul;28(4):566–73.

The Skin Picking Scale-Revised (SPS-R)

Instructions: For each item, pick the one answer which best describes the past week. If you have been having ups and downs, try to estimate an average for the past week. Please be sure to read all answers in each group before making your choice.
(1) How often do you feel the urge to pick your skin?
0 No urges
1 Mild, occasionally experience urges to skin pick, less than 1 hr/day
2 Moderate, often experience urges to skin pick, 1–3 hr/day
3 Severe. Very often experience urges to skin pick, greater than 3 and up to 8 hr/day.
4 Extreme, constantly, or almost always have an urge to skin pick
(2) How intense or "strong" are the urges to pick your skin?
0 Minimal or none
1 Mild
2 Moderate
3 Severe
4 Extreme

(3) How much time do you spend picking your skin per day?
0 None
1 Mild, spend less than 1 hr/day picking my skin, or occasional skin picking.
2 Moderate, spend 1–3 hr/day picking my skin, or frequent skin picking.
3 Severe, spend more than 3 and up to 8 hr/day picking my skin, or very frequent skin picking.
4 Extreme, spend more than 8 hr/day picking my skin, or near constant skin picking.
(4) How much control do you have over your skin picking? To what degree can you stop yourself from picking?
0 Complete control. I am always able to stop myself from picking.
1 Much control. I am usually able to stop myself from picking
2 Some control. I am sometimes able to stop myself from picking.
3 Little control. I am rarely able to stop myself from picking.
4 No control. I am never able to stop myself from picking.
(5) How much emotional distress (anxiety/worry, frustration, depression, hopelessness, or feelings of low self-esteem) do you experience from your skin picking?
0 No emotional distress from picking.
1 Mild, only slight emotional distress from my picking. I occasionally feel emotional distress because of my picking, but only to a small degree.
2 Moderate, a fair amount of emotional distress from my picking. I often feel emotional distress because of my picking.
3 Severe, a large amount of emotional distress. I almost always feel emotional distress because of my picking.
4 Extreme, constant emotional distress. I feel constant emotional distress and see no hope of this changing.

(6) How much does your skin picking interfere with your social, work (or role) functioning? (If currently not working, determine how much your performance would be affected if you were employed.)
0 None
1 Mild, slight interference with social or occupational activities but overall performance not impaired
2 Moderate, definite interference with social or occupational performance, but still manageable.
3 Severe, causes substantial impairment in social or occupational performance.
4 Extreme, incapacitating
(7) Have you been avoiding doing anything, going any place, or being with anyone because of your skin picking? If yes, then how much do you avoid?
0 None
1 Mild, occasional avoidance in social or work settings.
2 Moderate, frequent avoidance in social or work settings.
3 Severe, very frequent avoidance in social or work settings.
4 Extreme, avoid all social and work settings as a result of the skin picking/scratching.
(8) How much skin damage do you currently have because of your skin picking? Only consider the damage produced by the behavior of picking.
0 None (No skin damage from picking)
1 Mild (Slight damage in the form of small scabs, sores, scrapes, etc. Damage covers a very small area and no attempts are made to cover or treat the damage).

2 Moderate (Noticeable scars, scabs, or small open sores (< 1 cm in diameter)). Picking results in attempts to cover or treat the damage with in-home remedies (e.g., bandages, creams, ointments) that do not require the assistance of a physician.
3 Severe (Large scars, scabs, or open sores (>1 cm in diameter)), infected areas and/or noticeably disfigured skin. Picking results in extensive attempts to cover the damage and may require periodic treatment by a medical professional (e.g., prescription antibiotics, dermabrasion, etc.)
4 Extreme (Large open wounds or craters, frequent bleeding, large scarred areas). Damage may require extensive covering and medical intervention (e.g., plastic surgery, stitches, hospitalization, etc.).

Yale-Brown Obsessive Compulsive Scale (YBOCS)

The Yale-Brown Obsessive Compulsive Scale (YBOCS) assesses the severity of obsessive and compulsive symptoms over the preceding week, and comprises 10 questions (5 for obsessions, 5 for compulsions). Each question is scored on a Likert-scale with higher scores indicating greater severity:

0 = None / Definitely resists / Complete control / No time at all
1 = Mild / Much control / <1 hour per day
2 = Moderate / Moderate control / >1 hour per day but <3 hours per day
3 = Severe / Little control / >3 hours but <8 hours per day
4 = Extreme / Completely yields / No control / >8 hours per day

The total possible score for the YBOCS is 40. Each subscale can be scored separately to give the clinician a degree of severity for the patients' obsessions and compulsions. As a guide, cut-off scores are as follows for OCD severity: 8-15 mild, 16-23 moderate, 24-31 severe, and >32 extreme.

The questions can be summarized as follows:

Obsessions Subscale (questions 1-5)

1) How much time do you spend having obsessions each day?
2) How much interference does having these obsessions cause if your life?
3) How much distress do these obsessions cause you?
4) How much resistance do you put up when obsessions enter your mind?
5) How much control over the obsessions do you have once they enter your mind?

Compulsions Subscale (questions 6-10)

6) How much time do you spend engaging in compulsions each day?
7) How much interference does engaging in compulsions cause?
8) How much distress does engaging in compulsions cause you?
9) How much resistance do you put up when obsessions enter your mind?
10) How much control over the compulsions do you have?

Overall composition of YBOCS severity items included with permission from Dr Wayne Goodman. For a copy of the YBOCS and permission to use the scale please contact Dr Wayne Goodman (wayne.goodman@mssm.edu). Goodman WK, Price LH, Rasmussen SA, Mazure C, Fleischmann RL, Hill CL, Heninger GR, Charney DS. The Yale-Brown Obsessive Compulsive Scale. I. Development, use, and reliability. Arch Gen Psychiatry. 1989 Nov;46(11):1006–11.

Obsessive Compulsive Inventory—Revised

0	1	2	3	4
Not at all	A little	Moderately	A lot	Extremely

The following statements refer to experiences that many people have in their everyday lives. Circle the number that best describes **HOW MUCH** that experience has **DISTRESSED or BOTHERED you during the PAST MONTH.** The numbers refer to the following verbal labels:

1. I have saved up so many things that they get in the way.	0	1	2	3	4
2. I check things more often than necessary.	0	1	2	3	4
3. I get upset if objects are not arranged properly.	0	1	2	3	4
4. I feel compelled to count while I am doing things.	0	1	2	3	4
5. I find it difficult to touch an object when I know it has been touched by strangers or certain people.	0	1	2	3	4
6. I find it difficult to control my own thoughts.	0	1	2	3	4
7. I collect things I don't need.	0	1	2	3	4
8. I repeatedly check doors, windows, drawers, etc.	0	1	2	3	4
9. I get upset if others change the way I have arranged things.	0	1	2	3	4
10. I feel I have to repeat certain numbers.	0	1	2	3	4
11. I sometimes have to wash or clean myself simply because I feel contaminated.	0	1	2	3	4
12. I am upset by unpleasant thoughts that come into my mind against my will.	0	1	2	3	4

13. I avoid throwing things away because I am afraid I might need them later.	0	1	2	3	4
14. I repeatedly check gas and water taps and light switches after turning them off.	0	1	2	3	4
15. I need things to be arranged in a particular order.	0	1	2	3	4
16. I feel that there are good and bad numbers.	0	1	2	3	4
17. I wash my hands more often and longer than necessary.	0	1	2	3	4
18. I frequently get nasty thoughts and have difficulty in getting rid of them.	0	1	2	3	4

Index